P9-CET-269

Health to the People

Stories of Public Health, Preventive and Lifestyle Medicine,

and Medical Evangelism Training and Outreach,

Loma Linda, California, 1905–2005

P. William Dysinger, MD, MPH

with Dorothy Minchin-Comm, PhD

2007

Order this book online at www.trafford.com/07-1126
or email orders@trafford.com

Most Trafford titles are also available at major online book retailers.

© Copyright 2007 P. William Dysinger.
All rights reserved. No part of this publication may be reproduced, stored in a retrieval
system, or transmitted, in any form or by any means, electronic, mechanical, photocopying,
recording, or otherwise, without the written prior permission of the author.

Note for Librarians: A cataloguing record for this book is available from Library
and Archives Canada at www.collectionscanada.ca/amicus/index-e.html

Printed in Victoria, BC, Canada.

ISBN: 978-1-4251-3087-9

*We at Trafford believe that it is the responsibility of us all, as both individuals
and corporations, to make choices that are environmentally and socially sound.
You, in turn, are supporting this responsible conduct each time you purchase a
Trafford book, or make use of our publishing services. To find out how you are
helping, please visit www.trafford.com/responsiblepublishing.html*

*Our mission is to efficiently provide the world's finest, most comprehensive
book publishing service, enabling every author to experience success.
To find out how to publish your book, your way, and have it available
worldwide, visit us online at www.trafford.com/10510*

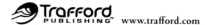 www.trafford.com

North America & international
toll-free: 1 888 232 4444 (USA & Canada)
phone: 250 383 6864 ♦ fax: 250 383 6804 ♦ email: info@trafford.com

The United Kingdom & Europe
phone: +44 (0)1865 722 113 ♦ local rate: 0845 230 9601
facsimile: +44 (0)1865 722 868 ♦ email: info.uk@trafford.com

10 9 8 7 6 5 4 3 2

About the front cover

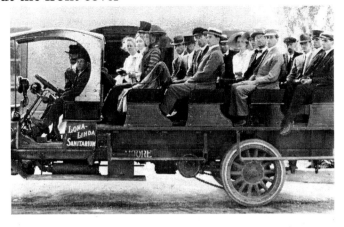

Then...   Medical Evangelism students and staff traveling to a community health education project near Loma Linda near the beginning of the 20th century.

Health to the People

*Stories of Public Health, Preventive and Lifestyle Medicine,
and Medical Evangelism Training and Outreach,
Loma Linda, California, 1905–2005*

... and Now!   CHIP graduation in Centerville, Tennesee, in February 2007. CHIP is the Coronary Health Improvement Project which LLU graduate Hans Diehl originated and which has become one of the largest and most successful community based lifestyle change programs currently available in the USA. This Centerville program was directed by Dr. and Mrs. P. William Dysinger, both Loma Linda graduates.

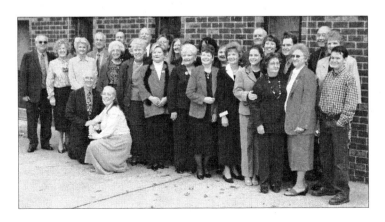

Table of Contents

Dedication

This storybook of Loma Linda public health history is dedicated to my dear wife, Yvonne Minchin-Dysinger, without whose love, encouragement, and direct assistance, I never could have completed this four-year labor of love. She has stood with me for more than 47 years and has been my principal support in raising our family of three boys—Edwin, Wayne, and John—and our daughter, Janelle. She has worked alongside me in nine years of missionary service in Cambodia, Tanzania, Singapore, Pakistan, and Yemen, and "held the fort" during much overseas work where I traveled and she remained at home. She has endured with grace our busy retirement years which have included, besides this book, the writing of another book and much work overseas as well as locally on our farm and near our home in middle Tennessee.

I would also dedicate this work to those committed pioneers on whose shoulders the current public health faculty and staff of Loma Linda University now stand. We must never forget the difficulties they faced and the courage with which they met and overcame problems that now make it easier to follow after them. When the way looked impossible it was simply an opportunity for those pioneers to exercise greater faith and work harder to train "medical evangelists" qualified to do medical missionary work in the places of greatest need in the world. Needs remain and their work is not yet finished.

Acknowledgements

I am very grateful for the support and encouragement I have received in the research and writing of this reference work. Special thanks go to Richard H. Hart, chancellor, and W. Augustus Cheatham, vice chancellor for public affairs; and Patricia Johnston, former dean, and Gordon Hewes, associate dean, School of Public Health, for assisting and encouraging the work from its beginning. Special thanks also goes to the Del E. Webb Memorial Library and its staff, especially to Merlin Burt (and his successor Michael Campbell) and the staff of the archives and heritage room where Yvonne and I spent many days and hours, and to the office of Lisa M. Beardsley, former vice chancellor for academic affairs and her secretary, Melanie Jackson. Each of the deans of the School of Public Health—Mervyn G. Hardinge, James M. Crawford, Andrew P. Haynal, Edwin L. Krick, Richard H. Hart, Patricia K. Johnston, and James L. Kyle II—have freely contributed. I am also anxious to acknowledge the great debt I owe to those who have otherwise contributed and/or have reviewed various parts of the manuscript and have given me corrections and suggestions that were needed and appreciated. These, among others, include Barbara A. Anderson, Steven Eric Anderson, Larry Beeson, Diane G. Butler, Terrence L. Butler, T. Allan Darnell, Albert Dittes, David T. Dyjack, Wayne S. Dysinger, Linda H. Ferry, Gary E. Fraser, Ella Haddad, Paul Hisada, Linda G. Halstead, Georgia W. Hodgkin, Joyce W. Hopp, Jayakaran Job, John H. Kelly, Synnove M. Knutsen, Jerry W. Lee, Naomi N. Modeste, Susanne B. Montgomery, Milton Murray, Christine M. Neish, Martine Y. Polycarpe, Raymond E. Ryckman, Joan Sabaté, Richard Schaefer, Teri S. Tamayose, C. Torben Thomsen, and Norman Woods. A very special thanks to Richard Weismeyer, his assistant, Carol Berger, and their staff for their extraordinary effort in helping to bring this book about.

Finally, special tribute goes to Dorothy Minchin-Comm for the magnificent contribution she has made in helping organize and otherwise edit this manuscript.

Preface

As I retired in 1992 after several years of government service and 35 years of working for the Seventh-day Adventist Church, one of the several things I had on my list to do was to help write a history of the School of Public Health at Loma Linda. I had been intimately involved, working with the founding dean, Mervyn G. Hardinge, in its beginning. As I quickly became involved in many other activities, however, I decided I would never get around to writing that history and put it completely out of my consciousness.

In 2000 my wife and I were in New Hampshire where we participated in the memorial service for Pastor J. Lee Neil and I mentioned there his contributions to the School of Public Health and especially to the restoration of lifestyle medicine in the Adventist Church (see Chapters 23–26). Afterwards, both his son and one of his daughters came to me with expressions that they had never before heard of their father's influence in these matters. It struck me forcibly that the pioneers were dying off and the accomplishments of their lives would never be recorded, or known, even to their own children, unless someone took the effort to research and record them.

Although still busy with other projects, I felt compelled to think again about seeking to recount the history, not only of the School of Public Health, but of all the public health entities and activities at Loma Linda from its beginning in 1905. I had tentatively written out a three page outline of such a history and was making plans to stop in Loma Linda, on our return from a mission trip to South Korea, to investigate the interest and support for such an effort. I was sitting at my desk at home in Tennessee one day in January 2001 with my history outline in front of me. I was thinking about how and who I should contact at Loma Linda regarding the history proposal when the telephone rang. I answered it and on the other end was Richard H. Hart, chancellor of Loma Linda University, calling to tell me the University administrators were planning for the centennial celebrations in 2005–2006 and recognized a need for a written history of public health at Loma Linda. "You have been selected to do the research and write the history. Are you willing to do it?" Hart asked.

Tears came to my eyes as I realized God had just performed another miracle of communication. Before I had communicated to Loma Linda, the University had communicated to me, answering all my questions before I had asked them. I was quickly reminded of a previous time when that had occurred back in 1974 (you can review this story on page 78). With the reassurance that God was in it and calling me, I consented to begin the task which has culminated in a reference CD and this book.

As I accepted the challenge, I assumed I would have access to all the correspondence files I left in Loma Linda and the minutes of the many administrative committees I chaired or attended. I looked forward to these documents refreshing my memory. Great was my disappointment when I discovered that all old files had disappeared. There is no evidence of any malicious destruction, but persons who did not recognize the value of the old documents no doubt rejoiced in their effort to clean out files. The lack of these records made my work very much more difficult.

To complete this task has taken many months of research in Loma Linda and almost four years of work otherwise. It has required research in the archives at the General Conference of Seventh-day Adventists, as well as at Loma Linda. To organize and substantiate this work required reviewing 100 years of University Board minutes, reading through all the Bulletins and other official publications of the University for the past 100 years—particularly the Medical Evangelist, the University SCOPE, the University Observer, and Today plus many other publications and books. It included interviews with dozens of persons who freely shared their stories and experiences. The results of this research are in this book and/or in the separate reference CD with the same title (see information box which follows this preface).

The intent of this storybook is to extract interesting stories and inspiration from the research. Each public health discipline is briefly described and illustrated in the history of community health and outreach programs from Loma Linda. I have sincerely tried to be as objective as possible in recounting events of historical significance. I have tried to be both concise and as complete as possible—a real oxymoron. A weakness is the fact that some people either seek and/or receive more publicity than others and I recognize very well that many who are never written up in University publications are just as worthy, or more so, than many who receive extensive publicity. I would very much like to honor the unsung heroes, but feel unable to do much more than what is in this book and its accompanying CD. I can only hope and pray that the excitement and drama of all that is public health will somehow come through in my feeble efforts.

Finally, I am much impressed by my review of history that God is alive and has worked marvelously through His human servants at Loma Linda during the past 100 years. It is truly wonderful to see how God has blessed and the many, many unique contributions Loma Linda has made to general public health education and for the promotion of health to many people around the world. I am almost overwhelmed by the recognition of what God can do through His human subjects if we can be more surrendered to His will. God is seeking to clearly illustrate His love in the lives of those who are ready to unselfishly serve others. Thank God for His representatives at Loma Linda and their demonstration of whole person care to the world. May balanced physical, mental, and spiritual health be so shared that His kingdom of peace might be quickly established. People need and are receptive to this type of health promotion.

P. William (Bill) Dysinger
Williamsport, Tennessee, USA
July 2007

About the "Health to the People" Reference CD

The reference CD about "Health to the People" is the equivalent of an almost 500 page book. It contains a great deal more detail than the story book, including many hundreds of citations. It contains a comprehensive time line of public health from its beginnings at Loma Linda and a roster that includes almost 500 of the public health professors who have taught at Loma Linda. It also contains a roster of 5,159 Loma Linda public health degree graduates from 1964 through 2003 and much other information that is not readily available otherwise. The CD is published in a searchable PDF format which enables any word or phrase to be found in the document. This reference CD can only be obtained at Nichol Hall, Room 1704, School of Public Health, LLU, Loma Linda, CA 92350. The access phone is (909) 558-4664 or fax number (909) 558-0845. The web address is: <www.llu.edu/llu/sph>. This story book is also available at the above addresses or through Trafford Publishing, <Amazon.com>, <Borders.com>, Barnes & Noble, and many other book sellers.

Foreword

More than 100 years ago, what is now Loma Linda University and Loma Linda University Medical Center began as a counter-culture movement among health care practices of the 19th century. Under the divine guidance of a small group of intrepid and firmly convicted pioneers, the institution laid out its operational mandates and began offering both health services and professional courses. The intervening century has seen that institution struggle severely at times, even questioning its purpose and mandate. But in the end, it has emerged as a world class university, known and respected in every country of this globe.

This book is the story of that journey, told carefully by one who has walked with the institution for many of those years. Bill Dysinger is an alumnus, a former administrator, and a longtime faculty member. His personal understanding and commitment to the original goals of this place are unquestioned. He has carefully dug through long buried archives and board minutes, talked with numerous individuals, and created the most complete story, ever told, of this aspect of the University. He recognized early on that this wasn't just a story of the School of Public Health, but rather a sometimes thin thread of philosophical commitment and professional empowerment that has been carefully nurtured from the very beginning.

As you peruse these pages, you will see the inside workings of a group of fallible individuals united by a common commitment to the greater good. They continually struggled with adapting to changing times while protecting our uniqueness. How well they succeeded is left up to the reader. But there can be no question of the divine origin and footprint throughout the history of this place. It is a message that must be understood and incorporated by our faculty, students, and alumni, even today.

From the early training of "Cooks and Bakers" to the current potpourri of academic degrees, the College of Evangelists migrated to the College of Medical Evangelists and eventually to Loma Linda University. At least part of the purpose of this book is to retell that history in an attempt to recapture the early fervor and commitment to simple remedies and health practices. While much of the world has now endorsed our health message, Loma Linda and the Seventh-day Adventist Church continue to provide the most balanced approach to both preventive and therapeutic health care today. Modern medicines and technologies have dwarfed some of those early modalities, but at the end of the day, the message of how to retain and regain good health is still a sought after message that is in our keeping. May this legacy be continued and enriched in the years ahead.

Richard H. Hart, MD, DrPH
Chancellor
Loma Linda University

Health to the People

1

The Sanitarium Idea

Traditionally, hospitals have existed for sick people. A blessed essential for the ailing multitudes, to be sure. The word "sanatorium" derived from the Latin sanatorius ("giving health") or sanare ("to cure"). In the 19th century, the word sanatorium specifically designated an open-air institution for treating the scourge of tuberculosis.

The "sanitarium" idea, however, went a long step further, indicating an institution for the promotion of health. Could people be trained to preserve their health and avoid the hospital altogether? Or, once stricken with disease, could they fight it with natural remedies instead of toxic drugs?

Apparently, John Harvey Kellogg coined the word "sanitarium" to describe the new Adventist institution at Battle Creek and to distinguish it from mental or tuberculosis hospitals. "That word," someone pointed out, "does not exist in the dictionary."

"Never mind," Dr. Kellogg replied confidently, "If it isn't there, it soon will be."

In Adventist circles, a "sanitarium" has always been a place for health education. A place based on a belief that what sick people need is a ministry to the whole person—body, mind, and spirit. Not by accident, sanitariums have traditionally been located in quiet, rural areas where patients can find serenity and sink into the heart of nature itself.

In 1876 Dr. J. H. Kellogg was made medical superintendent of the new Battle Creek Sanitarium. (The previous Western Health Reform Institute had been initiated in 1866). Here in Battle Creek a new concept of lifestyle and preventive medicine would be born.

As medical superintendent, Kellogg introduced treatments firmly based on the health principles advocated by the Seventh-day Adventist Church. Radiation therapy

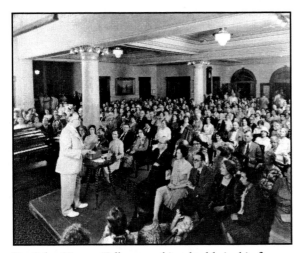

Dr. John Harvey Kellogg teaching health in his famous parlor talks at the Battle Creek Sanitarium. A "sanitarium" has always been a place for health education.

for cancer patients and the invention of flaked breakfast cereal were a couple of his innovations. His brother, W. K. Kellogg, carried the latter product into big business. His bold red signature may still be seen on cereal boxes on every grocery shelf.

Twenty years later, the idea of the "sanitarium" had truly arrived. Indeed, it had reached all the way to California. Up to this time, California had been "thinly populated." San Diego a drowsy military outpost. Los Angeles a hotbed of crime. When the Santa Fe Railroad thrust its way into Los Angeles in 1887, however, everything changed.

The Hill Beautiful

Surrounded by the highest mountains in Southern California (Baldy, San Bernardino, San Gorgonio, and San Jacinto), this beautiful inland San Bernardino valley charmed one and all. The lovely landscape, the fertility of the land, the perfection of the climate—who could ask for more? As railway ticket prices plummeted, people from the East and Mid-west poured into California, seeking health and prosperity.

Forthwith, a group of developers in Los Angeles published a promotional brochure describing "Nature's Great Sanitarium" in the idyllic San Bernardino Valley. They chose a little hill just south of the railway tracks and named it Mound City. For $40,000 they built an ornate, ultra-Victorian hotel atop the "mound."

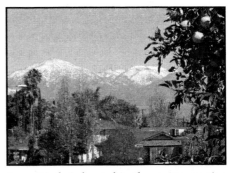

Loma Linda is located in the orange-growing San Bernardino Valley. This picture looks northwest from Loma Linda across the valley to Mount San Bernardino and San Gorgonio (aka "Greyback").

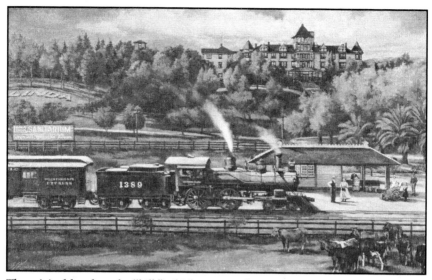

The original hotel on the "hill," which was transformed into the Loma Linda Sanitarium in 1905. The train station and the stairway up the hill are prominent in this picture. (This is a Nathan Greene painting on display in the lobby of Loma Linda University Medical Center.)

Barely was their project complete when a prolonged drought and a financial depression hit concurrently. The enterprise collapsed.

The Mound City group sold the land to a corporation for just $15,000. The new owners consisted of 40 businessmen and 80 physicians from Los Angeles. They zealously invested $155,000 into renovating the hotel and creating a health resort. Of the many such resorts springing up around them, they determined to make this the best of them all. They advertised widely and even ran excursion trains out from Los Angeles to acquaint people with the new facilities and amenities. A double line of tiered steps ascended from the Loma Linda train station to the hotel.

The owners changed the name from the unimaginative Mound City to Loma Linda, meaning "Hill Beautiful" in Spanish. To no avail. The business never prospered, and the promoters abandoned the old hotel on the mound. Even though the little Hill virtually floated on the fragrance of orange blossoms from the orchards all around, nothing helped. Instead, the Hill was waiting for something else. Some, in despair, called it "Lonesome Linda."

A Destiny Fulfilled

In 1904 the owners of Loma Linda decided to cut their losses and offered the property for $110,000. A marvelous opportunity! Sixty-four rooms in the hotel (with elec-

16

tricity), five separate cottages, a large recreation hall, fruit orchards, and farm buildings. Moreover, much of the 76 acres of land had been landscaped with lawns, drives, and walks. The deal also came with horses, cows, chickens, and turkeys, plus wagons, carriages, and farm implements. Another $12,000 worth of hotel furnishings would be thrown in. A real boon to this desert location was an artesian well with abundant water, a pumping plant, tower, and tank. The water had already been piped all over the property.

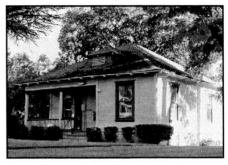

One of the original five cottages that came with the hotel. This cottage is now (2007) used as the office for SIMS.

A young pioneer pastor with good business acumen now appeared on the scene. Although John Allen Burden knew about the Loma Linda property, he also understood that the $110,000 price tag was wholly out of reach. Besides, during the previous year, two other sanitarium properties (Glendale and Paradise Valley) had been purchased in the Southern California Conference. This, at the behest of one of the Seventh-day Adventist Church founders, Ellen G. White. For a membership of just 1,000 in Southern California, the proposition had to be hopeless. Besides, they already carried a debt of $40,000 and the General Conference policy of "no debt" was being zealously promoted.

Then, the owners reduced the price to $85,000, soon followed by another drop to $45,000. These signs of desperation kept Burden on his toes, and the selling price finally bottomed out at $40,000.

Mrs. White immediately urged the purchase. "Secure the property by all means, so that it can be held, and then obtain all the money you can to hold the place. This is the very property we ought to have. Do not delay .... It's cheap at $40,000."

Meanwhile, the local conference officers were away at meetings in Washington, D.C. Torn between Ellen White and the negative views of the brethren, Burden had been soliciting funds. On May 25, he received $2,400 from a Los Angeles farmer. The next day he used $1,000 of this money to make a down payment. The sellers would give no further options.

At this time, a disturbing telegram came from Washington, D.C. to the Western Union office in Los Angeles. It advised: "Do not make deposit on Sanitarium." Signed: G. W. Reaser (president of the Southern California Conference). For reasons never understood, the telegram was delivered to the wrong person!

After returning from Washington, D.C., on Monday morning, June 12, 1905, everyone converged on Loma Linda to discuss the property. Since the $1,000 down payment was non-refundable, Burden could only hope and pray for the best. That day, Mrs. White and her son, Willie, arrived from the Redlands Railway Station in an express wagon. As she was shown through the buildings, she kept exclaiming, "I saw this before—four years ago!" She spoke of the educational work to be carried out here. "Battle Creek is going down. God will re-establish His work in this place."

In the afternoon, Ellen White spoke of gospel medical missionary work. "She spoke in a manner," John Burden declared, "that surpassed anything I ever heard her say." Among the listeners in the hotel parlor that afternoon were two significant visitors. One, the superintendent of the Mound City Corporation, said, "We wanted to do something we were not capable of. We know you people will carry out the plans."

The other, a previous owner of Loma Linda, cried, "Mr. Burden, I would give anything to be with you in this thing. This is what we wanted. We got some ideas from your folks at Battle Creek." Tears streaming down his face, he searched for words. "But no two of us could agree on anything we wanted, so we got into difficulty and had to sell out." Perhaps those 120 businessmen and physicians were doomed to failure by sheer numbers! The man ended his testimony simply: "I am so glad you have it."

To Have and to Hold

So far, so good. Now to pay the bill. With empty pockets and that debt of $40,000, how was the conference going to manage this thing?

Just a week after the site-visit to Loma Linda, John Burden and Ellen White attended a conference-wide constituency meeting in Los Angeles. Burden described the beautiful property that had fascinated him from the first time he saw it. Ellen White spoke at length about Loma Linda as a sanitarium. The conference president responded appropriately: "Sister White has said that this sanitarium should be the principal training school on this [West] coast."

A stir behind him, and the president heard a firm, familiar female voice: "This will be." Delegates from the 22 local churches overwhelmingly voted "Yes."

Everyone went home in high spirits, leaving John Burden to figure out how to raise the $40,000. As things stood, he had to add $4,000 to his initial down payment by early July. He did this by means of much, much effort and many, many small gifts. Three more payments of $5,000 each would come due in August, September, and December. The remaining $20,000 had to be paid in three years.

On the day when the August payment came due, John Burden didn't have a single penny in view. The pessimists feared that the conference credit would be jeopardized. "Better we lose the $5,000 than go ahead," they cried. "Don't you see that we face an utter impossibility?"

Others stuck by Ellen White's words and refused to declare failure. Tension mounted on both sides. Then, in the midst of the argument, the contenders heard the postman coming up the stairs. "For you." He put a letter into the hand of the conference president.

In the envelope? You guessed it. A draft for $5,000! The exact amount needed for the payment that day. Then another amazing circumstance came to light. The letter had been postmarked in Atlantic City, New Jersey, two weeks earlier.

Eyes filled with tears. One of the severest nay-sayers broke the silence: "It seems..." his voice trembled, "that the Lord is in this matter."

"This time was solemn as Judgment Day," another would remember. From that day forward the spirit of criticism disappeared.

By marvelous—sometimes miraculous—circumstances the entire debt of $38,900 was removed before the end of 1905. Happily, the prompt payment provided a much appreciated $1,100 discount.

Those long-ago men and women of faith and fortitude would be amazed to see what their original sacrifice has produced. Today Loma Linda University has a state-of-the-art Medical Center and a strong program in teaching health science. With assets now exceeding one billion dollars, Loma Linda's efforts in public health, lifestyle and preventive medicine, and other outreach have had a very significant global impact.

Explaining how and why these wonderful things came to be will occupy the rest of this book. Specifically, how the health emphasis and community outreach developed at Loma Linda.

2

Two Lengthened Shadows

S o there the Hill Beautiful stood, ready to serve. A plan for the school still had to be formulated. With few precedents to look to, confusion would inevitably prevail at the start. Of the many stories told of the founding of Loma Linda University, we must limit ourselves to a few.

When Ralph Waldo Emerson wrote that "every institution is the lengthened shadow of one man," he hit upon a great truth. In the case of Loma Linda, however, we must consider the "shadows" of two people, Ellen G. White and John Allen Burden. These two stand out as the designers of the plan to make Loma Linda a health-training center.

Ellen Gould White (1827–1915)

The life of Ellen White has already been widely documented. An earnest Christian girl in the Methodist church in Gorham, Maine, she and her family entered heartily into the Adventist Millerite religious revival of the early 1840s. At age 17 she experienced the first of the some 2,000 visions she would have during her long, seventy-year ministry to her Church. Along with it came the instruction to "make known to others what I have revealed to you." Over the years she would write a phenomenal number of books, along with thousands of tracts and periodical articles, plus another 60,000 pages of letters, diaries, and other manuscript materials.

In 1846 Ellen Gould Harmon married James White, an early Adventist evangelist. Only two of their four sons would survive to adulthood. Both Ellen and her husband struggled with poor health. Then came one of the most pivotal messages of her entire career, an extensive vision on health reform. She received it in Otsego, Michigan, on June 6, 1863—just two weeks after the Seventh-day Adventist Church had been officially organized.

This comprehensive revelation covered the entire range of health and preventive medicine. The causes of disease and the care of the sick, nutrition and remedial agencies, the dangers of narcotics and stimulants, child-care and sensible dress. All of this called for the obligation ("sacred duty") of each person to give intelligent attention to the health of body and mind.

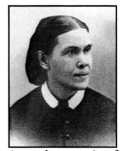

Ellen White struggled to fulfill her own recommendations. A heavy meat eater, she scorned the simple, wholesome foods that she, under inspiration, had recommended. "Serve us no more meat," she instructed her cook.

An early portrait of Ellen G. White, an important founder of the Seventh-day Adventist Church. She was the prime instigator for the purchase of Loma Linda.

Promptly, at the next meal, Ellen faced a table bountifully laden with good food but completely bare of meat. The cook followed her directions to the letter. Ellen took one look at the prepared meal, however, and left the dining room. Good and hungry, she hurried to the table for the next meal. Again, she turned away, painfully aware that the only food she craved was flesh food.

At the third meal, Ellen stared at the food with disgust. Crossing her arms, she severely announced: "Stomach, you may wait until you can eat bread." She, of course, won her battle with appetite, but vegetarianism was but a small fragment in the far-reaching implications of the new health reform.

With her husband, James, Ellen White crossed the American continent many times, forwarding the interests of the infant Adventist Church. After James' death in 1881, she spent two years in Europe, followed by nine years in Australia. Finally, in September 1900, her ship docked back in the United States—in San Francisco. This 72-year-old lady did not know where to make her next home.

Two enticements led her to consider the West. Proximity to the Pacific Press, in Oakland, California, was convenient for her writing and publishing needs. Secondly, she had a passionate interest in developing new sanitariums in Southern California.

Next came a frenetic search for a place to live. When she saw the house of the railroad builder Robert Pratt in St. Helena, she knew she had come home. She bought the 60-acre farm with its fully furnished, seven-room house for $5,000. She named it "Elmshaven," after a row of elm trees in front of the house. She moved in, just 25 days after she had disembarked from the ship from Australia.

Such a brief sketch cannot do justice to this diminutive little woman—5' 2", dark complexion, brown hair, and gray eyes. Cheerful, unselfish, and outgoing, she was known as a careful housewife, a sensible buyer, a hospitable hostess, a forceful public speaker, and a good neighbor. Her profound otherworldly interests notwithstanding, she followed all of the local news and could enjoy a good laugh.

Although she never accepted a formal leadership position in the Church, Ellen

White's voice came through loud and clear in matters of health education as well as many other Adventist concerns. The only governing board on which she agreed to serve was that of the self-supporting institution at Madison, Tennessee.

John Allen Burden (1862–1942)

John Burden grew up to believe unwaveringly in the inspired counsel of Ellen White. She had the message, and he managed the money—and much more beside. Born in a log cabin in Grant County, Wisconsin, he was only nine years old when he went to an Adventist meeting. He joined the church at twelve. By 1882, John Burden had enrolled in Healdsburg College in Northern California.

From the start of his career, Burden became enmeshed in medical missionary plans and management, beginning at the St. Helena Sanitarium. There, as manager, he met and married Eleanor, the bookkeeper.

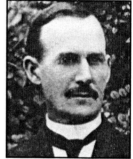

John A. Burden was a firm supporter of the inspiration that came through Ellen G. White. He took a leading role in raising the funds for the purchase of Loma Linda and was the principal organizer of the beginnings of CME.

As Mrs. White departed from Australia, the Burdens went down under to work in the new Sanitarium, just north of Sydney, New South Wales. After four years spent there establishing the medical interest, the Burdens returned to California. The "Lady of Elmshaven" now wanted them to promote sanitarium work in Southern California.

In January of 1905, John Burden had led out in the purchase of Glendale Sanitarium. By the end of that same year, through a chain of providence, he had completed the purchase of Loma Linda. Throughout those amazing months, Ellen White urged him to get the school open for training "medical evangelists."

In December 1915, the Burdens moved from Loma Linda to Paradise Valley Sanitarium, just south of San Diego. John served as business manager there, until his wife died in 1934. He spent his last years back at the Hill Beautiful, always ready to field questions about God's leading in the founding of the College of Medical Evangelists.

On a June evening in 1942, Burden, having just finished giving a Bible study, was walking home in the dark from Redlands to Loma Linda. A car struck him, and he died instantly. J. L. McElhany, president of the General Conference, preached the funeral service on June 14. Burden is buried next to his wife in Chula Vista, California.

No matter what the circumstances, John and Eleanor Burden never disregarded Mrs. White's counsel on health reform—or on any other belief, for that matter.

They could not, however, foresee the long procession of years that would pass in the slow growth of public health and preventive medicine ("health to the people") on the Hill Beautiful.

Among all of the many founders of lifestyle medicine, Ellen White and John Burden together cast a very long shadow indeed.

3

Making a School from Scratch

The Seventh-day Adventist Church had taken possession of the Loma Linda property on July 1, and the first patient registered on October 12, 1905. No working capital existed, and no one had any assurance they would receive a salary. Nonetheless, by November 1, 35 staff members were on duty. By Christmas that year, 25 patients were comfortably lodged in the new sanitarium.

In April of the next year, Mrs. White again came south, this time with Elder and Mrs. Stephen Haskell from New England. She intended that they should teach and sponsor evangelistic activities. They all participated in the April 15 dedicatory service of the "Loma Linda Sanitarium." Lunch followed an inspection of the buildings and grounds, the meal bespeaking its Southern California context. Oranges mingled with sandwiches made of nuts, fruit, egg, and olives; cake, jelly-roll, and cereal coffee followed.

The program for the afternoon session featured four speakers, the last being Ellen White. She eloquently charged the audience to open a training center for "medical evangelism." Although the College of Evangelists, as it was first called, officially opened on September 20, 1906, instruction did not actually begin until October 4.

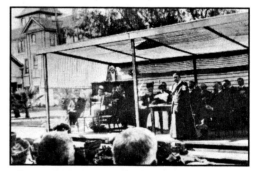

Ellen G. White was the principal speaker for the dedication of the Loma Linda Sanitarium and its training programs on April 15, 1906.

The early administrators could agree on at least some definitions, but others aroused confusion. The word college indicated a center of education. No problem there. Evangelism meant sharing the "good news" of the gospel with others. Medical evangelism had to refer to telling the public that God wants to help humankind move towards restoration of his original perfect health. Defined by soundness of body, mind, and spirit, health, then, includes more than just the absence of disease or disability. (The World Health Organization subscribed to this new definition as it was founded in 1948). The confusion on the Loma Linda campus reigned primarily in defining "medical evangelism" and the details of teaching plans and curriculum to reach that objective.

The Southern California Seventh-day Adventists based their project solidly on Scripture: God's desire is for more than just spiritual health. "Beloved, I pray that you may prosper in all things and be in health, just as your soul prospers" (3 John 2). God's Word also proclaims that, "if anyone defiles the temple of God, God will destroy him. For the Temple of God is holy, which temple you are" (1 Corinthians 3:17). Thus, violation of nature's laws becomes a moral problem. "Therefore, whether you eat or drink, or whatever you do, do all to the glory of God" (1 Corinthians 10:31). This suggests God is interested in a total and very comprehensive definition of health and good health practices. In keeping with Heaven's policy of free choice, however, people's participation in lifestyle changes is strictly voluntary.

Putting the Pieces Together

As manager of the embryonic institution, John Burden faced the challenge of creating an "evangelistic-medical course." The training, of course, would conform to Ellen White's injunction: "Thousands of workers are to be qualified with all the ability of physicians to labor, not as physicians, but as medical-missionary evangelists." It would, however, take decades of effort—and, yes, conflict—to understand and try to implement this inherently paradoxical statement.

During the first school year (1906–1907) five women enrolled as freshman "medical students." At the same time, they were also listed as senior nursing students. In this manner, health education training began at Loma Linda.

Formulating a curriculum called for Burden's best skills. Aged 43, with 14 years of sanitarium work behind him, he became the chief mentor of Loma Linda education for the next 10 years. Additionally, he chaplained the Sanitarium and brought together a small Adventist congregation on campus. He assembled four courses, designed to train two types of workers: nurses and medical evangelists (public health educators).

Not surprisingly, nobody seemed to know exactly what the evangelistic-medical course should be. Moreover, church administrators still had to figure out exactly how it would fit into the organized work of the Church.

The third college prospectus in 1909 admitted that the school was not "as yet" prepared "to grant the usual medical degree." That idea, however, clearly lay just

---

Courses Offered in the 1906–1907 School Year at Loma Linda

1. Nurses Course (three years)—allowed for the last year to cover the first year of the evangelistic-medical program.
2. Evangelistic-Medical Course (three years)—designed for graduate nurses and others interested in advanced medical studies.
3. Collegiate Course—a special program for those wishing to experience sanitarium work before continuing to other college studies.
4. Gospel Workers' Course—a field-training program intended to be a constituent part of each of the foregoing courses.

---

under the surface of the institution's thinking. Meanwhile, people were encouraged to come and work in a "strong medical missionary setting" that advocated treating disease by "simple, natural means."

Burden hoped that the training would appeal to "well-trained nurses." Hopefully, many of these would attain the "ability of physicians" but still be willing to work as evangelists. Finally, a few "fully accredited physicians and surgeons" had to be found to take a leadership role in these ambitious enterprises.

John Burden never lost sight of the goal for "strong scientific course" blended with a "strong evangelistic and Bible course." Even he, however, could not possibly foresee all the complexities to come.

The Balance Tips

Under the laws of the State of California, the school was chartered on December 9, 1909, as the "College of Medical Evangelists." Loma Linda's medical school evolved in 1910 with the addition of two clinical years to the existing three-year medical-evangelistic course. The administration limited enrollment only to those who wanted to do "the work of the Christian physician and medical missionary."

"We have no time to devote to merely giving a medical education to those who wish to practice medicine," the faculty proclaimed. "This certainly is no time for Seventh-day Adventist young people to seek a training for the ordinary work of a doctor."

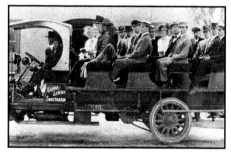

Medical missionary outreach was, from the beginning, very important at Loma Linda. Here a truckload of medical evangelists heads out into the community.

High purpose notwithstanding, medical evangelism as a separate training entity rapidly fell into a decline. During the next fifteen years, the three-year course shrank to two years and then one year. At last, it faded into oblivion as a three-month program. By 1926 interest in the non-degree program was so little that no such health education training was offered anywhere at the College of Medical Evangelists. The initial health education training had skidded to a halt. The highly desirable MD degree won out. By 1928, CME had become the largest medical school in the western half of the United States. Now, the challenge of accreditation would loom over Loma Linda for years to come.

Still, questions lingered. The General Conference president, A. G. Daniells, wondered—in 1913—whether they had made a mistake in establishing a full-fledged medical school. After all, they had been conducting a medical missionary school successfully.

Considering the nearness of the Second Coming of Jesus, Dr. C. W. Flaiz asserted that "men needed to go out quickly into the field and bring men to the knowledge of the truth." Indeed, in 1914, he proposed that better results (that is Christian conversions) might be had from the languishing three-year evangelistic course than from the five-year medical degree.

CME administrators like Drs. Newton Evans and Percy T. Magan continued to mourn the loss. Great effort, much money, and wide-spread advertising had failed to bring in evangelism students. The young people (understandably) were wont to say: "If we get this training, we are not preachers, we are not nurses, and we are not doctors. We are nothing, and we have no degree."

A few enrollment statistics from the early years reveal the medical school consistently overshadowing the training of medical evangelists. Having begun in 1906 with five students, the medical-evangelistic course reached its maximum enrollment of 45 in 1916. It steadily declined to zero in 1925–1926. Recruiting good students became increasingly difficult and the drop-out rate ran high.

In contrast, the medical school began with an enrollment of 10 in 1910, most transferring directly from the medical evangelistic course. By 1927 CME had 372 medical students—the largest enrollment of any medical school in the western United States.

Not one to despair, Dr. Magan appealed for reform in 1926. He declared: "Before the end of time, every good word that God as ever spoken concerning this place will be fulfilled." Somehow, medical ministry would have to unite with preaching the gospel.

Long experienced in sanitarium work, Dr. J. H. Kellogg offered little comfort. "Doctors," he told Magan darkly, "are high-headed people." He could see no way to retain the graduates in medicine within the ideal of medical missionary endeavor.

Finally, against the tide of opposition, Magan concluded, "So we dropped the effort."

It would be another 40 years before a serious revival in health evangelism training would be attempted at Loma Linda.

4

The Nuts and Bolts
of Medical Evangelism

The career of one of the earliest and most prominent practitioners of medical-evangelism must be coupled with that of a member of the last CME "medical evangelism" class to demonstrate the diversity and the range of grass-roots experience.

A Pair of Pioneers

Although John H. N. Tindall came from a Methodist home in California, the doctrine of hell-fire so deeply offended him that he became an atheist. While studying law in San Diego, he detoured to join a gold strike near the Mexican border. There he met one he called "a man of mystery." That person read to him from the writings of Ellen White, leading Tindall from the "gold field rocks" to the "Rock of Ages."

Forthwith, the school year of 1908–1909 found Tindall as one of eleven "Bible and Special" students at the College of Evangelists. Shortly, he and his wife became active in making a practical application of Ellen White's health-reform vision in 1910.

Willmonte D. Frazee (1906–1996) finished in the last medical evangelism class in 1925. At 17 he and his brother Titus (aged 16) had come to Loma Linda in 1923 when their mother began teaching elementary school there. Having only home-schooling behind them, the teenagers' application baffled the faculty. Whatever made the boys think they could enroll in the medical-evangelism course? The boys were admitted to the "adults only" course on a trial basis. "You will receive no credit," the teacher warned. "And you must not, on any account, hinder the other members of the class."

Bill Frazee reveled in Dr. Alfred Shryock's classes in anatomy and physiology and scored 100 percent on the final test. From this point onward, he could take any courses he wished. Happily, he created a mixed bag of medical evangelism for himself. Taking two years of the nursing course, and advanced chemistry, he went on to choose what he liked in the dietetic curriculum.

The second year, Frazee took more chemistry and joined the dietitians for another year of physiology. By this time, his teachers were urging him to take the medical course and become a "proper" doctor. He based his refusal on Ellen White's appeal not "to spend years in preparation," because gospel medical missionaries "are needed now."

Among Frazee's classmates was the veteran medical evangelist, Elder John H. N. Tindall, who had returned to CME to take the non-degree dietetics course (1924). This additional knowledge, he asserted, would enable him to reach many otherwise unapproachable men and women "of the higher classes." Tindall and Frazee became laboratory partners and studied together. The weary, older man appreciated the tutorial help he received from his bright, younger companion.

The men bonded. When Tindall chose Frazee to assist him in the establishment of his Field School of Health Evangelism in San Francisco, the conference officers became suspicious. Bill Frazee had qualified neither as a minister nor as a health worker. The brethren could have spared themselves the anxiety. Following Tindall's example, Frazee conducted many successful campaigns in California, Utah, Arkansas–Louisiana, and elsewhere. He later started the training institution in Wildwood, Georgia where a new concept of lifestyle medicine was pioneered.

Team Work Pays Off

During the night of February 27, 1910, Ellen White was shown new ways to carry out medical evangelism. She spoke particularly of the "unworked cities." For this mission, she called for "companies (teams) to be organized and diligently trained to labor in our important cities." Although he had not finished any specific health course, Elder Tindall was chosen to try out the new medical-evangelistic methodology in a pilot program. He set up in nearby San Bernardino.

He faced a struggle, for his wife had not yet become an Adventist. They had a very young baby, and she was less than enthusiastic about the arrangement. Her husband would be totally immersed in the campaign for six weeks. One of the college teachers, Charles Garnsey, and his wife, Margaret—both nurses—joined the team.

They pitched their tent next to a building where a prominent ladies' club met. Overhearing one of the health talks, the president invited Tindall to address her club. Having thus gained access to influential city leaders, he rejoiced when the editor of the San Bernardino newspaper gave the Adventists much advertising space, gratis, through editorials and full page reports of the meetings.

A wealthy businessman who attended the meetings recognized that he was on the verge of becoming a Seventh-day Adventist. He could not, however, give up his tobacco. Because of a heart condition, he thought that giving up the habit would kill him. Tindall assigned the nurses to give him special attention. In an example of a team effort, through their ministry and prayer, he eventually got the victory. Thrilled with the outcome, the man announced: "I'm just going to stick that old pipe up on a post in my backyard. It will remind me of the idol that almost killed me." (Later, the grateful, now-healthy man made an interest-free loan of $10,000 to Loma Linda at a time when that institution very much needed the money).

At the end of this pilot program in San Bernardino, 16 people were baptized, Tindall's wife included. The results electrified Loma Linda. Suddenly, the cities had become a viable mission field. Thereafter, Tindall became a full-time medical evangelist and went on to other campaigns elsewhere.

Oklahoma City (1920)

Tindall's usual work plan involved the gathering up of a team of "paid conference workers." They included the evangelist and his assistant, Bible workers, doctors, nurses, a singing evangelist, and cooks. Then he organized local church members to give Bible studies and simple treatments. They also distributed announcements and ushered at the meetings. Always skilled at public relations and community involvement, Tindall interviewed prominent business firms and asked for contributions. Furnishings, groceries,

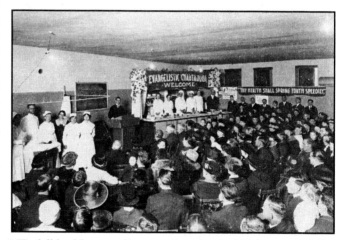

A Tindall health evangelism team in action in Oklahoma. Tindall is at the pulpit in the center.

laundry work, utensils, and more came in. Since all of these things were donated, the health evangelistic work became as self-supporting as possible.

Tindall always secured the largest, best-equipped auditorium in town. Then, he rented a smaller hall to accommodate treatments and cooking classes. Three meetings convened each week:

1. Tuesday. A lecture on the optimum diet.
2. Thursday. A discussion of common diseases, their prevention, causes, symptoms, and treatment.
3. Sunday. A strong, stirring gospel message. (Tindall concentrated on three gospel themes: the seventh-day Sabbath, the nature of man, and the Spirit of Prophecy (writings of Ellen White).

In Oklahoma, to everyone's surprise, the audience of 1,700 swelled to more than 2,000, after the Sabbath question had been presented. When the popular evangelical preacher Billy Sunday arrived in town, many predicted a greatly decreased attendance at Tindall's meetings. After all, Billy Sunday had the support of major city officials as well as the leading newspapers. Amazingly, the audiences at the Adventist lectures continued to increase. At the last meeting, 500 people stood to indicate their belief in the messages presented. "Billy Sunday got the crowds," someone remarked, "but Tindall got the converts."

All in all, these exciting results allayed much prejudice against Adventists. Conference workers had received good training for their future work, and church members had savored a new, exhilarating sense of service. Financially, the campaign had carried its own weight and had stimulated a faithful tithe income. Above all, people flocked into the church—and not just temporarily. Months later "every new convert" had been "thoroughly instructed in every doctrine [and] every reform in physical, mental, and spiritual habits." Perhaps the most significant result of Tindall's medical-evangelism approach proved to be the solid long-term establishment of people "in the faith."

Much gratified, the Oklahoma state medical secretary declared: "If other religious people would do as practical a work [as Tindall], it would be a great help to people everywhere."

A Roster of City Team Work

From the Mid-West to the West Coast, the "Tindall Method" of medical missionary work put down its roots in many places. In 1921, Elder Tindall conducted a Medical Missionary Training School in Dallas, Texas. Fifty representatives from Seventh-day Adventist Churches and the Southwestern Union Conference attended his lectures. The deep and lasting impact not only changed personal habits, but also fired up a zest for soul winning. In that day of meticulous record-keeping, members reported weekly on their "hours of Christian help work and number of treatments given." The brethren also tallied up how many articles of clothing had been donated and kept account of the quantity of tracts distributed. Well pleased, the administrators reported that all of these activities had increased four-fold after the Tindall effort.

Another example of Tindall's innovative health education projects took place in Redlands, California (1921–1922). The evangelistic campaign, of course, contained a strong health component. As the nutrition lectures went on, he announced an unusual demonstration. Two chickens were lodged in the front window of a nearby grocery store. They would be fed different diets. The first one ate only whole wheat bread. The other, white bread. In a short time, the white-bread "subject" began to deteriorate. She showed symptoms of Vitamin B deficiency and suffered from neurological abnormalities.

The show stirred up the interest of the town and brought down the wrath of the Humane Society. (This from people who consumed chicken at dinner at least every Sunday!)

Just before her demise, however, the poorly fed hen was given whole grains. She made a dramatic recovery, and the sale of whole wheat bread in Redlands, it is said, increased mightily.

John Tindall's field school in San Francisco (1927–1931) proved to be the largest evangelistic training effort ever undertaken by a CME medical evangelist. The school year divided into three trimesters of 16 weeks each. The subjects involved 688 hours of Bible and evangelical studies and 576 hours of health and medical training. Monday morning staff meetings brought all students and staff together to review progress and discuss problems. More than 100 medical evangelists completed the program. Among them was J. Lee Neil, who would later have much influence in the Loma Linda health program.

Meanwhile, Bill Frazee had opened up his own field school in Ogden, Utah (1931). His staff of 29 included 8 graduate nurses, a physician, a chef, and a singing evangelist. In this time of depression, however, only the evangelist and his assistant received a salary. The rest volunteered. Public lectures on "health and efficiency" preceded the main campaign.

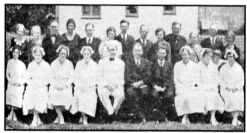

Frazee's large team for his field school of health evangelism in Ogden, Utah, 1931.

These were given in high schools and to other groups throughout the city. Home nursing and cooking classes were taught, and house-to-house visitation occurred. This extensive outreach resulted in positive public recognition and 15 free minutes on the local radio station, three times a week.

Frazee always paid tribute to the quality of his training at Loma Linda. He made good practical use of this blend of scientific principle and Bible truth. "I see how fully they meet the needs of the poor, sick world." Ultimately, he pioneered the concept of "conditioning" or lifestyle change when he founded a training institution for health evangelism in Wildwood, Georgia.

5

The Business of Eating

Historically, in ancient and more primitive times, eating was a matter of finding enough food to be strong and to stay alive. The encroachments of "civilization," however, have consistently overturned the balance between the products of the earth and the creatures that must use them. The distortion seems to go back to the Garden of Eden when the Serpent used food to deceive Eve. Ever since, affluence and appetite, plus the disparities between supply and demand, have turned eating into a "business"—and a problematic one at that. Over eating is the bane of Western culture, to be sure.

An investigation of nutrition in the Middle Ages is an exercise in astonishment. How could people eat that way and survive? Actually, they didn't. In many places life-expectancy was as little as 25 years. In the early 19th century, however, some experimental work began on the diets of children and criminals.

In 1870 Dr. Pavys wrote a treatise on foods and dietetics. As a result, interest in England arose and many schools of cookery sprang up. At the same time, a French professor of gastronomy came to America with his Italian cook. They toured the large Eastern cities with lectures and demonstrations. Then, having established the New York Cooking Academy, they returned to France.

The aftermath of this novel enterprise encouraged physicians in both Boston and Philadelphia. The latter group hired Mrs. Sarah Tyson Rorer to establish a diet kitchen where they could prepare special orders for specific patients. Interest in the science of food and cookery, as well as diet therapy, took a long leap ahead and never turned back. The Medical School of the University of Pennsylvania helped to pioneer this new dietetic service.

In 1908 a small group of women interested in hospital dietetics founded the American Home Economics Association. It languished until 1917 when the soon-to-be influential and powerful American Dietetic Association (ADA) first came into existence with a charter membership of 58.

The Adventist Edge

The Seventh-day Adventist Church, however, pre-dated these health interests by more than 50 years. Ellen White's instructions in 1863 had been taken seriously, as exemplified in Dr. John Harvey Kellogg's work and his teaching at the sanitarium in Battle Creek, Michigan.

Not surprisingly, from the first year of operation (1906), Loma Linda College of Evangelists inserted "domestic science" into the nursing course. "Medical dietetics" followed in the second year. Indeed, "hygienic cookery" became part of all nurses' training, and they practiced their arts in a diet kitchen, serving both the sick and the well.

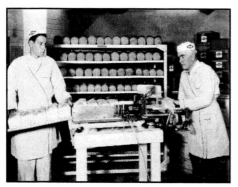

The cooks and bakers course began at Loma Linda in 1908.

By 1908, the College had sufficiently established itself to be able to make a serious announcement. The new "cooks and bakers course" would train "competent hygienic cooks and bakers." This new initiative promised to be "very thorough in practical work and heavy in studies." Only those "willing to work hard" should apply. Moreover, limited facilities would reduce each class to no more than 10 students. Graduates would receive a diploma to confirm their qualifications. By 1912, the one year course had been reduced to nine months. The beginning of World War I terminated it altogether, but not before other planning for dietetic training had started.

In 1922 Dr. E. H. Risley (dean of the Loma Linda campus of CME) delivered a thought-provoking discourse to the Adventist General Conference session, reviewing the latest science in nutrition. His paper on "The Newer Dietetics" paved the way for the beginning of nutrition education in September of that year in Loma Linda.

The two-year course would train dietitians for hospitals and other institutions, as well as promote both church and public lecture work. Surely, the time had come to formalize the education of the people who would implement

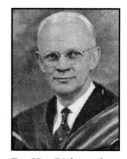

E. H. Risley, dean of the Loma Linda campus of CME, laid the groundwork for the establishment of dietetics training.

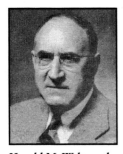

Harold M. Walton, the first male member of the American Dietetic Association, was the first dean of the School of Dietetics.

the ideals that the Church had held for so many years. Formerly a dietitian at St. Helena Sanitarium and the first male member of the American Dietetic Association, Harold M. Walton became the first dean of this new school at Loma Linda.

By 1930, the School of Dietetics raised its entrance requirements from twelve to fourteen grades of schooling. The two "pre-dietetics" years (provided by all Seventh-day Adventist colleges at the time) would enable a student to graduate with a four-year BSc degree (major in foods and nutrition and a minor in chemistry).

In one way, the years of World War II presented a golden opportunity for dietitians to share the Adventist health plan. Such popular commodities as meat, sugar, and coffee, so important to many, were rationed. Della Reiswig describes her experience in Los Angeles. Elder Folkenberg, pastor of the Los Angeles Central Church, secured the comfortable, beautifully equipped, spacious diet kitchen attached to the large basement auditorium of the Southern California Gas Company for a cooking school. This vegetarian school had an average attendance of 200. On a Tuesday evening in March the attendance greatly increased. As the air raid siren shrieked and all the employees in the large building filed in, Della learned that she was teaching in the designated bomb shelter for that building. During the hour before the "all-clear" signal sounded, very many learned the principles behind "Victory Meatless Meals" who would never have been reached otherwise. The war time was a golden opportunity for health reform teaching.

As World War II intervened, however, applications to the dietetics program began to fall off. Moreover, Loma Linda's dietetic internship training was not yet recognized by the American Dietetic Association. A financial squeeze had begun, and trouble reared its ugly head. In desperation, some suggested a major effort to encourage young ladies "to take up the study of dietetics." By 1948, however, those

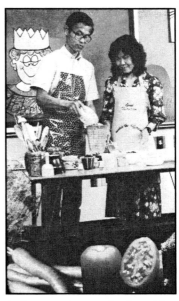

An important outreach of nutrition has always been cooking schools. Here, Dr. and Mrs. Clarence Ing are shown presenting a cooking school to the public.

recommending the closing of the School of Dietetics at Loma Linda became louder in their demands. Others debated the proposition of leaving nutrition to the Seventh-day Adventist colleges, with Loma Linda providing only a dietetic internship.

The announcement of the closing of the collegiate program in nutrition at Loma Linda came in 1953, and the axe fell in 1954—when all current students had been able to complete their work. Between 1922 and 1954 CME graduated 244 dietitians in the nutrition program, either from the diploma program or the bachelor's degree.

Salvaging the Fragments

The College of Medical Evangelists without a nutrition program? How could that be? The problem of accreditation had arisen once more. As dean of the School of Dietetics in the early 1930s, Dr. Risley knew that anyone wishing to become a registered dietitian had to have credentials from an accredited school. CME's accreditation with the American Medical Association would not do for dietetics or nursing.

Forthwith, dean Risley pressed forward with his quest for accreditation and recognition by the American Dietetic Association. (Perhaps it is well that he could not foresee that the process would take more than 20 years).

To initiate accreditation, Dr. Risley personally presented CME's application to the Northwest Association of Secondary and Higher Schools in April 1937. That Association voted favorably and announced that "the College (CME) has been given full accreditation." (The Western Association of Schools and Colleges, LLU's current accrediting body, did not come into being until 1962.)

With general accreditation in hand, it was now time to organize an internship approved by the American Dietetic Association. A long series of hindrances began with the first ADA assessment in 1939. The inspectors made two recommendations. Dietitians needed at least three months of administrative experience in a dietary department. Second, they had to have a one-month affiliation to gain "intensive meat experience." That is, to learn the grades and cuts of meat as well as meat cookery.

In order to meet the demands for the next inspection in 1944, a huge effort was made to find dietitians who were ADA members. Ruth Little was persuaded to leave Paradise Valley Sanitarium and move to White Memorial Hospital on CME's Los Angeles campus. Nonetheless, the next inspection also failed. The nonplussed Board of Trustees finally uncovered the hang-up. The ADA announced in April 1945 that it could not accept CME's teaching and practice of vegetarianism.

After years of further effort, appeals, and many inspections, finally, in 1958, Dr. Ruth Little was able to announce that the accrediting body had "unanimously approved" CME's dietetics internship and its new MS degree program. Twelve years later the dietetic internship moved to the Loma Linda campus. Its survival was no longer threatened.

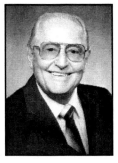

The doctoral research of Dr. Mervyn Hardinge at Harvard University in 1952 began cutting a swath through the field of public opinion. His was the first effort to make a good comparative study of vegetarians and non-vegetarians. He studied lacto-ovo-vegetarians, pure vegetarians (vegans), and non-vegetarians (as controls). Significantly, he found that a lacto-ovo vegetarian diet is not inferior to that of the non-vegetarian. Dr. U. D. Register had already helped pioneer research on vitamin B-12 and was the first chair of the department of nutrition in the School of Public Health.

U. D. Register was the first chair of the department of nutrition in the SPH. Dr. Kathleen Zolber joined the University as director of food service at the LLU Medical Center in the late 1960s. She led the way in developing a coordinated undergraduate and internship program in dietetics (ADA approved in 1972). The impetus continued as Lydia Sonnenberg chaired an ADA committee to a write a position paper on "The Vegetarian Approach to Eating." By now, the dietetics program was divided between the Schools of Public Health and Allied Health Professions.

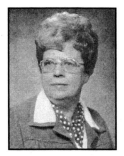

Shortly after, three Loma Linda professors (Register, Zolber, and Sonnenberg) wrote ADA's manual on vegetarian diets, "The Vegetarian Diet, Food for Us All." The ultimate irony occurred in 1982 when Dr. Zolber, a Loma Linda vegetarian professor, was elected to the presidency of the then 50,000-member American Dietetics Association, the organization that had for twenty years disapproved Loma Linda and its vegetarian diets. She was later awarded the Cypher Award, ADA's most prestigious.

Kathleen Zolber was director of dietetic internship at Loma Linda and became president of the 50,000 member American Dietetic Association.

From Rags to Academic Riches

Nutrition knowledge increased and, after long frustration on all sides, vegetarianism entered the mainstream. The large International Congresses on Vegetarian Nutrition organized by Loma Linda faculty have had a major impact. These congresses convened in 1987, 1992, 1997, and 2002, with the proceedings fully reported in special issues of the highly acclaimed *American Journal of Clinical Nutrition.*

In 2003 the latest issue of the *Loma Linda University Diet Manual* was published, a 950 page handbook edited by Dr. Georgia Hodgkin. It is now a tremendous vegetarian resource for all Adventist hospitals. Many other medical institutions such as Harvard, Yale, and Stanford have also found the book extremely valuable.

The current (2007) chair of the School of Public Health's department of nutrition, Dr. Joan Sabaté, originally a physician from Spain, edited *Vegetarian Nutrition, A Public Health Approach* (2001) that has become the definitive textbook on vegetarianism. He and his colleagues tracked nutritional epidemiology and studied data from the Adventist Health Study. One of their findings concerned nuts. Eating nuts related to decreased atherosclerosis and coronary heart disease. Walnuts topped the list, but since then almonds, pecans, and even the lowly peanut have attained scientific stature. Today Loma Linda and Dr. Sabaté, among other things, are the recognized world experts on the health effects of nuts. Indeed, Loma Linda is internationally celebrated for the nutrition teaching and research of its faculty.

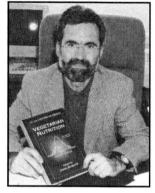

Joan Sabaté is chair (2007) of the nutrition department of the SPH and is shown here with the textbook on vegetarian nutrition which he edited.

What's So Great About Vegetarianism?

Health reform did not wholly begin with Ellen White. The founder of Methodism, John Wesley (1703–1791) proclaimed great health truths. When liquors and wines were common household commodities, he advised total abstinence. His fiery zeal also denounced tobacco, tea, coffee, and condiments and he promoted vegetarianism. He was followed by Dr. Sylvester Graham (1795–1851), a Presbyterian clergyman who waged war against refined cereals. To him we owe graham (whole wheat) bread. Founded by the Congregationalists in 1833, Oberlin College, Ohio, produced very strict reformers. All flesh food was forbidden, along with pies, puddings, rich pastry, tea, coffee, and condiments.

Almost concurrently, Ellen White began to learn the elements of health reform. Today her principles have been correlated and corroborated by science and have risen far above their early label of "fads." Her description of a good diet has often been quoted: "Grains, fruits, nuts, and vegetables constitute the diet chosen for us by our Creator. These foods, prepared in as simple and natural a manner as possible, are the most healthful and nourishing. They impart a strength, a power of endurance, and a vigor of intellect that are not afforded by a more complex and stimulating diet" (1909).

Nutrition and diet became the subject of profound research by the beginning of the 20th century. Unfortunately, the Adventists were not as good at marketing their health reform diet as some others. The Battle Creek entrepreneur, Charles Post, for instance, influenced a thousand to drink his cereal coffee, Postum, while the Seventh-day Adventist's might have persuaded one drinker to give up tea and coffee. W. K. Kellogg very successfully promoted breakfast cereals as an alternative to bacon and eggs. It is unfortunate that sugar-laden cereals have now lost their original healthful identity, and are now more closely related to cookies and candy than healthy breakfast cereals. Crass commercialism, one might cry. Whatever the motive, however, the success must be acknowledged.

Meanwhile, in CME classrooms teachers were giving advice at least 75 years ahead of their times. "One great error being made today by practicing physicians," Dr. W. D. Sansum declared, "is their neglect of diet. Some of us feel sure that one half of all human ills are due to improper diet .... The most essential error in diet in the United States today is the lack of fruit and vegetables. As a nation we must get back to the use of these natural foods" (1924). This was decades ahead of current nutrition recommendations to eat "five or more fruits and vegetables each day."

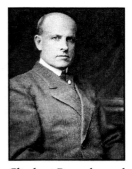

Charles Post learned healthful nutrition at Battle Creek and successfully marketed his cereal drink, Postum, and other breakfast foods.

An early CME medical evangelist, Julius Gilbert White, achieved practical results in Sacramento in 1925. He presented "the very simplest things we can find in the old 'health reform' message." A leading bakery in town began making 100 percent whole wheat bread to supply the demand created by his health talks. Eventually, they were selling 250 loaves a day where previously there was almost no demand.

Presently a dark little secret was uncovered. The dairy and meat industries had for many years manipulated university departments of nutrition with large dona-

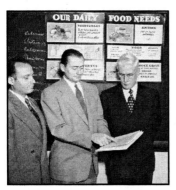

U. D. Register is shown here presenting a report to Harold N. Mozar (left) and Francis D. Nichol (right). Nichol is the one for whom Nichol Hall is named.

tions. Obviously, their encouragement would be toward using "complete proteins." People had to consume meat and dairy products to protect their health. In the 1950s, however, research turned up a disturbing fact. Saturated fat and cholesterol (almost entirely from animal products) became linked to the primary cause of death in the United States, atherosclerosis and coronary heart disease.

During his post-graduate study at Harvard University (1961–1962), Dr. P. William Dysinger encountered an excellent professor of nutrition, Dr. Jean Mayer. In a class on the history of public health, Dysinger literally witnessed the end of the strangling influence that the meat and dairy industries had over the science of nutrition.

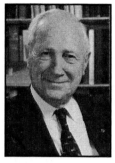

Jean Mayer was a Harvard professor of nutrition who chaired the First White House Conference on Nutrition and later became president of Tufts University.

Originally from Paris, France, Dr. Mayer had migrated into a distinguished career in nutrition at Harvard University, Massachusetts. In 1962, CBS television had launched a series of one-hour documentaries on important subjects. A documentary the previous evening on heart disease featured the celebrated Dr. Mayer from Boston as a world expert on serum cholesterol. He gave his scientific opinion on the relation between diet and heart disease.

Mayer was immediately followed by representatives of the meat and dairy industry. "Don't worry," they soothed. "Just forget about the so-called dangers of too much cholesterol in your blood. Just remember that you need protein from meat and dairy products in your daily diet."

The next morning in class, Dr. Mayer erupted in a rage. "They said that the cholesterol problem is just a passing fad." Sputtering as he went, Mayer outlined the shocking history of the "arranged marriage" between the meat industry and many university departments of nutrition. "Well, today," the professor exclaimed, "we have come to a parting of the way. Scientific nutrition cannot listen any longer to biased information from an industry dependent on the sale of its animal products."

From where we stand now, no one would dare say that cholesterol "doesn't matter."

Why Be a Vegetarian?

Vegetarianism has come into its own, at last. The reasons for accepting it, however, are diverse. One popular motivation concerns animal rights and the suffering of animals in today's "farm factories." Another rises out of Asian religious traditions (Hinduism, Buddhism, and Jainism). Concerned with the sanctity of life, these adherents had to make space for their belief in the transmigration of the soul.

Powerful ecological arguments for vegetarianism have arisen. The statistics can really stop traffic! Forty percent of the world's grain goes to feed animals for the meat market. Were these grains consumed by humans directly, five times more people could be fed. When land production is no longer sufficient, it was assumed the world could always turn to the sea for food protein, but increased world population and fishing actually drove the fishing industry to its limits back in 1989. With an absolute shortage of foods comes an ethical question. "Is it right for wealthy people in the world to 'waste food' by eating animal products, while so many others perish from malnutrition and starvation?"

For Loma Linda University, however, the impetus toward vegetarianism harks back to its early Adventist beginnings. Health benefits are now known to be enormous: fiber, vitamins, minerals, antioxidants, and phytochemicals come almost entirely from plants. Plant diets are proven to reduce heart disease, cancer, diabetes, and many other degenerative diseases. These things have been on Loma Linda's agenda for a long time.

To top it off, Adventists believe that they have a moral obligation to care for the bodies that God has given them.

6

Real Life Preventive Medicine

Health education, carefully prepared courses, field training, accreditation, research, funding. Within the limitations of those early days, CME had carefully tended to all of these things. The testing of these endeavors lies, of course, in real life changes in people. We offer two case studies. Two little women, barely 5 feet tall, migrated across the Canadian border and came to Southern California. Both became internationally known exemplars of what good nutrition and healthy lifestyle can really do.

Hulda Hoehn-Crooks (1896–1997)

Hulda Crooks is the most publicized and best known Loma Linda dietetics graduate and employee of the School of Public Health. Her biography, *Grandma Whitney, Queen of the Mountain*, was published just the year before she died.

Her parents migrated from Russia and homesteaded in Saskatchewan, Canada. She and her three brothers grew up on the prairies where farm living dictated a heavy meat and dairy diet. Added to that, Hulda spent her days snacking on peanuts, soft-centered chocolates, and chewy caramels. That "privilege" came with long hours of clerking in the family's country store. By the time she was sixteen she was carrying 160 pounds on her petite 5' 2" frame.

Hulda and her brother Ed set their sights on higher education. Seeing no particular need for book-learning, their parents left the teenagers to work their own way through an academy in North Battleford, Saskatchewan. One of the first Adventist schools in Canada, it was situated directly on the east-west fur-trapping route between Winnipeg and Edmonton, Alberta. There at Battleford Academy, Hulda and Ed Hoehn met Samuel Crooks, and all three of them graduated together in

1920. Although long hours of work at 18 cents an hour left little time for study, they somehow survived. Together, they headed for Southern California. Ed and Sam prepared to become physicians.

Hulda began training in dietetics at Loma Linda. Three months into her studies she succumbed to influenza, followed by pneumonia. After she returned much later to her classes, she always felt tired. When he was in his junior year of medicine, her fiancé, Sam, learned that he had high blood pressure and an enlarged heart. In October 1927, Hulda and Sam married "for better or worse." Health-wise, neither bride nor groom was worth much. Still, the "better" lasted for more than 20 years. Sam started as an instructor in anatomy (at $29 a week), eventually becoming chair of the department at Loma Linda and a nationally known anatomist.

The "worse," however, lurked in the corners of their minds as Sam's tired heart continued to weaken. Knowing she could lose him at any moment, Hulda often thought about life without him and frequently slipped into despair. One night, near the end of August 1950, she awoke with a start. Remembering one of Sam's favorite sayings, "We must go to the wild to keep from going wild," she saw her way ahead. She would go into nature to learn lessons of strength, fortitude, and serenity. From her kitchen window, she could see the highest mountain in Southern California, San Gorgonio, 11,500 feet high. Excitedly, she told Sam about her "call to the wild." Before dawn the next morning, she was on the trail, climbing her first peak, San Gorgonio. "Dear God," she prayed, "help me to keep climbing, whatever happens." A sweet joy filled her heart as she returned to the trailhead where Sam waited for her.

Hulda found her path to survival none too soon. Five days later, Sam fell victim to his final, long-expected heart attack.

Another dark cloud had also been shadowing Hulda's life. Their only child, Wesley, had fallen victim to alcohol and other drugs. A month before his father's death, he announced that he was married and that he wanted to enter medicine. This he actually did, graduating as a physician at UCLA. Three wives and three children later, however, his personal life was a shambles. His dependency problems had caught him in a revolving door of self-destruction. It spun faster and faster, until he died of a drug overdose in October 1969.

As a bereaved wife and mother, Hulda Crooks had truly thrown herself into the healing arms of nature. Two years after Sam's death she began working as a research associate of Dr. Mervyn Hardinge, the founding dean of the School of Public Health. For the next thirty-five years she wrote for numerous scientific publications. Her excellent professional achievements notwithstanding, Hardinge regarded Hulda's greatest contribution as a "remarkably humble and godly woman" who had the "ability to take the things of nature and bring out spiritual lessons." (These gems have been preserved in the book *Hulda Crooks: Conquering Life's Mountains*). She always enjoyed campouts with University students, who appreciated her wit, humor, and knowledge of Southern California's flora and fauna.

Hulda's mountaineering achievements brought her all the way to Congress (she climbed to the top of the Capitol dome at age 90), to the White House, and beyond. Her story appeared in local newspapers, numerous health publications, and TV shows. After a crew from NBC joined her in the three-day, 11-mile journey to the summit of Mt. Whitney, she appeared on Johnny Carson's "Tonight Show." Also, "Good Morning, America," "Games People Play," and more.

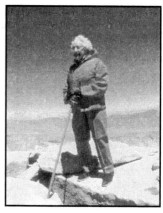

Hulda Crooks on top of "her mountain," Mt. Whitney, the tallest in the continental United States, 14,495 feet. She climbed it annually from age 66 until age 91.

Having climbed San Gorgonio some twenty times, the 66-year-old hiker was invited in 1962 to try 14,495 foot high Mt. Whitney, the highest mountain in the continental United States, for the first time. For the next 20 years she made it to the top of Mt. Whitney every year (1962–1982). She did miss one, but she made up for that by conquering Whitney twice in 1968. Indeed, she, along with everyone else, came to regard this one as her mountain.

Beginning at age 81 (1977–1987) Hulda, with a select hiking group and an experienced guide, climbed 90 of the 268 Southern California peaks listed in the Sierra Club Registry—most of them 7,000 feet and above. At age 91 she broke all records by climbing Mt. Fuji in Japan and "her" Whitney for the twenty-third (and last) time. These records brought enormous publicity to her commitment to maintaining physical, mental, and spiritual health.

Congressman Jerry Lewis had long admired Hulda's agility and her fondness for Mt. Whitney. "I'd love to do something like that some day," he confided to Hulda.

"Then you should do it," she replied. "But you need to lose some weight first." Gently, the white-haired great-grandmother nurtured him, as he swam, lifted weights and shed 30 pounds." Finally, she pronounced him fit. "We'll do it to celebrate my 90th birthday!"

Lewis declared that she had totally changed his life. Her every "spoken word exuded love" and every action was a physical reminder that "one is never too old to pursue a healthier lifestyle."

Thoroughly fired up, Lewis persuaded Congress to make a rare exception—bestow an award on a living legend. On August 21, 1991, an Army Chinook helicopter carried Hulda, Congressman Lewis, and some of her friends to the 12,000 foot high trail camp of Mt. Whitney. "I really don't know why I'm coming up here," she murmured. A big surprise awaited her.

There she met many of her friends and relatives who had hiked up the trail to

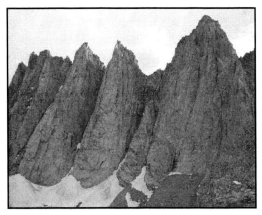

Mt. Whitney is the peak on the right; Crooks Peak is the second peak to the left (south) of Mt. Whitney.

meet this 95-year-old icon. Jerry Lewis began reading the congressional proclamation: "The second peak south of Mt. Whitney, the highest peak of Pinnacle Ridge shall be known and designated as Crooks Peak."

Hulda spun around to face the cheering crowd. Then she laughed, and laughed, and laughed some more. "This is beautiful! Just beautiful!" Next followed greetings from President George H. W. Bush, former President Ronald Reagan, and California Governor Pete Wilson. Until the end of time, 14,240 foot high Crooks Peak will stand as a granite testimony to the courage and spirit of Grandma Whitney who climbed until she conquered. Surely, Sam Crooks would have been proud.

The late Peter Jennings, ABC's anchorman, summed up the life of his fellow-Canadian well. "Mrs. Crooks has only one passion and that is her health …. At 18 with very little education, she left the farm and moved to California where the Seventh-day Adventists taught her the value of diet and exercise." Forthwith, Jennings named her on July 24, 1987, as ABC's "Person of the Week."

A New Kind of Ministry

Her healthful lifestyle and vegetarian diet were, at grass roots, a physical consideration. Hulda Crooks, however, turned them into a marvelous ministry. In fact, she prepared a little pamphlet, "A Prescription for Health," to give to people she met on the mountain trails.

Her writings abound in pithy bits of advice: "When all of your organs work efficiently, your brain (the most vital organ of all) will make intelligent decisions for you." "Use a regular exercise program, but work toward it gradually." "Have regular hours for sleep, rest, and relaxation." "Don't underestimate the power of mental attitudes. Anger, jealousy, hatred, wounded pride, anxiety [and much more] sap your life forces." "Be grateful for what good comes to you, be it ever so little." "Talk of things that give you joy." Ultimately, "health will be your prize for living in harmony with the laws established by your Creator."

In her later years Hulda Crooks lived in her apartment at Linda Valley retirement home. This amazing little person died exactly in the way you would expect—peacefully in her sleep at 101 years of age.

Another Canadian

Mavis Minchen-Lindgren (1907–2003) came from Kelowna, British Columbia, Canada. She is the poster-girl for all of the lay-people who catch the vision of the possibilities of lifestyle medicine and (literally) run with it.

Mavis had always had a predilection for chest problems. She had whopping cough at two, tuberculosis at thirteen, and unnumbered chest colds for most of her life. She took nurse's training at Rest Haven Hospital, Vancouver Island, British Columbia, but she met her husband, Carl Lindgren, at home in Kelowna. First and foremost, he was a lab technician with interludes as administrator of hospitals and nursing homes. They had three children: Kelvin, Mauvoreen (Muffy), and Karen.

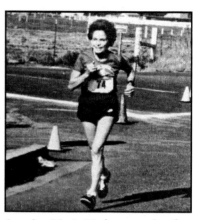

Amazing Mavis Lindgren ran her first marathon at age 70 and continued as a competitive runner until age 90. Her exercise overcame her severe respiratory disabilities.

By the time she was sixty-two, Mavis had become the typical, retired (sedentary) senior citizen. Then she came home from the hospital after her fourth bout of pneumonia in five years. "I am sick of being sick," she announced. "I'm going to make some changes." As a nurse, she well knew that penicillin was not the answer to her woes. She also received inspiration from School of Public Health professor Charles Thomas' fitness enthusiasm.

So she started running. Just as simple as that. She never had another cold. Never, one might ask? "Well," she admitted sheepishly. "I once had a real bad dose of flu. It lasted for three hours."

With a world-wide health consciousness developing all around, Mavis Lindgren quickly evolved into a well-known figure. She picked up headlines like "Five Miles a Day Keeps the Doctor Away," and "Great Grandma in Running Shoes," and organizations like Blue Cross of America used her for their advertising.

One observer said that Mavis looked like "the little old lady people want to help across the street." At one scant inch over five feet, she weighed just under 100 pounds. She did not, however, need help crossing the street.

At first she ran her races in a dress. "But, Mother," her daughters remonstrated, "people will think you're running away from home and get scared."

The ever conservative Mavis went next to slacks. Finally, she donned a regular running costume. Why not? She had a figure that women one-quarter her age could envy, so the short-shorts looked fine. Along with the girls, her physician-son took great pride in her accomplishments, as did husband Carl. After a race, she amazed everyone by how fast her "come-back" time could be. Her high complex carbohydrate vegetarian diet helped restore her muscle glycogen levels for the next race.

At age 85, "amazing Mavis" was tested and found to have an oxygen capacity equivalent to women 58 years younger than her. Her body fat composition was 12 percent compared to the average middle-aged woman who has 32 percent body fat. Her breathing capacity was 40 percent above predictions for her age, an amazing statistic in light of her former lung problems. Once an elderly overweight woman with lung problems, she seemingly threw off the limitations common to age, and ran her way back to the "fountain of youth."[1]

Although Mavis did not run marathons until the time that she died at age ninety-four, she did come close, completing her last race at age 90. For some twenty-five years, she showed up in races in far-flung places: Honolulu, Hawaii; Ottawa, Canada; Sacramento, California; Eugene, Oregon; and many, many more.

Actually, these two little expatriate Canadian women in Southern California had been friends from girlhood. Hulda was earning her school expenses by selling Adventist books among the scattered Saskatchewan farms. She traveled by horse and carriage. In Swan River, a wheel broke while she was at the Lindgren place. The men repaired the wheel and sent her on her way, but not before Hulda had told them a great deal about the Seventh-day Adventist Church.

After joining the Church, the Lindgrens moved to Kelowna, British Columbia, in order to provide their children with a Christian education. Mavis married Carl there, and the rest is history. Hulda and Mavis corresponded through the years. Although Mavis never climbed Mt. Whitney and Hulda never ran a marathon, the two were comrades in the practice and promotion of healthful living.

[1] David C. Nieman: *The Adventist Healthstyle*, Review and Herald Publishing, 1992, pp 119–122.

7

The Mission of Environmental and Tropical Health

B y its title alone, environmental health would appear to be a major concern of public health. People often misunderstand, however, the intermediary term "tropical medicine." They assume that this label must refer to diseases occurring in hot climates.

Nothing could be further from the truth. For example, Hansen identified Hansen's disease (leprosy) in his laboratory in Bergen, Norway. Leprosy posed a very real problem in northern Norway in the 19th century. In the 15th century more than 1,400 "lazar houses" (leprosariums) existed in France. Former president of the United States James K. Polk died of cholera in Nashville, Tennessee, in 1849. So many waves of cholera from South Asia and the Middle East swept through Europe and on to the United States, that international controls had to be established. The first International Sanitary Conference convened in Paris in 1851. High on the agenda were the cholera, plague, and yellow fever epidemics scourging Europe. In the 18th century even malaria raged through Boston and the rest of Massachusetts. Recently, amebiasis (an intestinal parasite) was a serious problem for the Eskimos in northern Canada.

In short, what we call tropical disease relates primarily to poverty and poor sanitation rather than proximity to the equator. Coincidentally, of course, many poorly sanitated developing countries are in tropical climates. Tropical disease control is basically an effort to improve environmental health.

Two Pioneers in the Field

From the start many CME graduates went to work in tropical areas. As early as 1910, Loma Linda offered medical students a short course in tropical medicine. Unfortunately, it proved to be limited and not very well organized. Most missionary physicians felt the need to study at Tulane University, Louisiana, or attend tropical medicine institutes in England or elsewhere in Europe.

The surge of interest in tropical medicine initiated by World War II forced the College of Medical Evangelists to take this phase of health care more seriously. During World War II, Dr. Harold N. Mozar (CME '36) found himself in the United States Army. He was assigned first to the Army Medical School in Washington, D.C., and then the University of Sydney, Australia. His military training was to prepare him to organize and direct an Army school of tropical medicine in New Guinea. Later, he worked in public health activities, both civilian and military, in the Philippines.

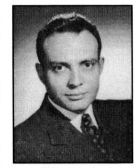

During his time in the South Pacific, Mozar recognized the great potential his tropical and public health experience had for augmenting the work of his church. Public health methods could influence masses of people, in contrast to the limitations of private medical practice. Training in prevention would have far-reaching health benefits. Preventive medicine could break the endless therapeutic cycle of sickness-treatment-sickness that left patients struggling like hamsters on a wheel. In their quest for better qualified instructors in preventive medicine, CME wisely secured Mozar's services for their faculty.

Harold N. Mozar, director of the Loma Linda School of Tropical and Preventive Medicine and trainer of missionaries in health education and tropical hygiene.

Meanwhile, a young medical student, Bruce W. Halstead (1920–2004), had enrolled at CME. Coming from San Francisco City College, he held an associate degree in biology. Since his early interest was in fish, he became a research assistant in the department of ichthyology at the California Academy of Sciences in Golden Gate Park (1935–1943). By the time Halstead reached Loma Linda, his interest in tropical medicine and public health had already started.

In his sophomore year in medicine, he really enjoyed a course in parasitology, taught by Dr. Gilbert Curtis (CME '39). It appeared, however, that teaching this topic was "one of their [the pathologists'] minor painful duties," the irrepressible Halstead declared. "I did not detect any real enthusiasm for the subject by the teaching staff."

In a practical test to identify Entameba histolytica (the cause of amebic dysentery) Halstead found that several of the slides had been identified wrongly. He went to the professor to make his point and to discuss the way parasitology ought to be taught in the medical school. "It was a stupid thing to do, but I also made some disparaging remarks about how the course was being handled."

Fortunately, Curtis took the criticism graciously. After all, this young man was top of the class. "If you think I don't know much about parasitology, why don't you come back to the school and teach the course?"

"Well, if the school will have me, I will," Halstead replied promptly. By the time he reached his junior year, he had an even bigger idea. Church statistics impressed him. CME was associated with an enormous network of mission stations: 6,000 foreign operations in 200 countries, 896 languages and dialects, 370 schools, and 219 medical institutions. Many of these were scattered in some of the most inaccessible tropical areas of the world.

After transfer to CME's Los Angeles campus, medical student Halstead visited the CME president, Dr. Walter Macpherson, and brashly announced, "Dr. Curtis has invited me to join the faculty and teach parasitology and tropical medicine."

Startled, the president reviewed the resume the young man had pushed across the desk. "Well, I agree that this does seem to be a good idea."

"There's more," Halstead went on. "I think CME needs a school of tropical medicine. Not only do I need a place to teach parasitology but I also want to set up a department of medical zoology. For my work in poisonous fishes and other marine organisms, you see."

Macpherson leaned back and smiled at the bold young medical student. "You know, you aren't the only one to have that idea. There's a Dr. Harold N. Mozar who served in the Army as a malariologist. He's also trying to start up a School of Tropical Medicine." The president smiled at Halstead's eagerness. "You two ought to get together." Scribbling down a number, he pushed a scrap of paper across the desk "Here's his phone number."

Combined Forces in the Cause

Halstead and Mozar's acquaintance began on the telephone and then extended into a long series of meetings. In 1946 the two submitted a proposal which was approved by the CME Board of Trustees. The next year, Harold Mozar, with the help of a $5,000 grant from Pacific Press, joined the CME faculty, full time. Plans went forward, and he became the first director of the School of Tropical and Preventive Medicine (STPM). That summer, ministers and missionaries took a new course in health education and tropical hygiene, the first formal training of missionaries by the Adventist Church.

From the beginning, the problem of finances reared its too-often-ugly head. Sensing the broad scope of the plan in relation to the Church, the General Conference discussed the proposition for three consecutive years (1946–1948). "The approval for the STPM," Mozar sighed, "came reluctantly." The brethren could justify the expenditure only if "the school would be partially self-supporting." Full of confidence and conviction, Mozar agreed.

The "charter" for the new school featured two main purposes: (1) to provide appropriate instruction in preventive medicine for doctors and other workers going to warm climates, and (2) to assist mission stations with their sanitation problems and, "where possible," help them to initiate community health programs. From the beginning, Loma Linda's School of Tropical and Preventive Medicine (the second such institute in the United Stated of America) intended to go far beyond the usual tropical medicine training institute. Mozar liked to remind everyone that "preventive medicine was from the beginning a part of our name."

Fresh from his internship at the Marine Hospital of the U. S. Public Health Service, San Francisco, Bruce Halstead arrived back in Loma Linda in 1947. He taught parasitology (as planned) and a tropical disease course for undergraduate nursing students. He really enjoyed teaching. The following year Halstead became assistant director of the STPM.

Funds, however, were desperately short. Courage and hope increased in 1949 with $25,000 from the estate of Mr. Robert Newbold. He earmarked the money for "the development of a school of tropical medicine in the College of Medical Evangelists." This fortuitous event occurred because of the donor's son, Dr. Robson Newbold (CME '44-A), who was in mission service in the Belgian Congo, Africa. Having taken the tropical public health training at Tulane University (1947), Dr. Robson wrote, "The subject of tropical medicine, for the first time in my medical studies, gave me a world-wide outlook …. It was the ideal course to increase my desire to serve in a foreign field." Therefore Robson Newbold persuaded his father to make this special bequest to CME to help begin a school of tropical medicine. The vision strong and the money essential. Good! A reliable, long-range financial system for the School, however, was yet to come.

8

Paying for the New School

The cheerful committee action that authorized the establishment of the School of Tropical and Preventive Medicine in 1948 included a new recommendation. A public relations department should be set up to relieve the Church of "a portion of the financial burden" involved with operating the new STPM. It should also cover expenses arising from "the normal expansion of the School." Moreover, this remarkable department should provide funds that would "contribute to the best interests of the medical work of the denomination as a whole."

For the first time in the history of the Adventist Church, a fundraising department was established within an Adventist institution. In addition to the mandate to raise all capital funds and miscellaneous expenditures, the General Conference agreed to appropriate $30,000 annually to support CME's new School of Tropical and Preventive Medicine and its missionary training.

In the first year, however, two untoward events transpired. The first General Conference appropriation turned out to be only $5,000. (It increased at the same rate per year until the $30,000 was reached in 1952). "The earliest money from headquarters," Mozar explained, "did no more than meet the debts accumulated during these fruitless years." Fruitless because all early attempts to obtain outside grant money had failed.

A Man for the Hour

In 1949 a well-qualified man stepped into this financial "sink-hole." Milton Murray had just graduated from La Sierra College with an English major and an interest in journalism and public relations. Wishing to serve the Church, he searched for employment with the publishing houses, schools, or medical institutions. Now he had reached a point of utter discouragement. Actually, he was asking his Church for a job that really didn't exist.

At the same time, Providence was at work, bringing two key men together. No Adventist college, at the time, offered majors in either journalism or public relations. Therefore, Dr. Halstead's efforts to find someone to start the new job at STPM had not yet succeeded. Rumors about the kind of man CME was looking for spread around La Sierra College. As Halstead talked to campus people there, one name kept surfacing. Milton Murray. "He's dynamic, a good salesman, and he gets along well with people. Moreover, he's fluent in both English and Spanish."

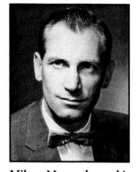

One Sunday morning on the La Sierra College campus Halstead tracked Murray down. "I'm Dr. Halstead from Loma Linda." The men shook hands. "Would you be interested in talking to us about being a public relations person for the School of Tropical and Preventive Medicine?" It appeared to be a "marriage made in Heaven."

Negotiations began. True, Mozar and Halstead had been "allowed" to organize a School of Tropical and Preventive Medicine (STPM) within CME. Arguably, the new institution could boost sagging faculty research at CME. Indeed, the accrediting association was reported to have been "singularly unimpressed with the faculty publication record at the medical school." This public relations

Milton Murray began his career as an internationally known PR leader and philanthropic fundraiser in the Loma Linda School of Tropical and Preventive Medicine.

person could put the new unit before the public and attract funding for research.

The project, however, faced more trials. Murray recalls that "The administration at Loma Linda didn't really understand the meaning of 'Public Relations.' So they were certain that they didn't need it."

After much debate, the executive committee made a bold, grand move. Murray would be hired for four months, but for the first two months only half-time. No point rushing into such a dangerous commitment! Nonetheless, ever the optimist, Murray accepted the appointment as a godsend.

Now he had a chance to prove himself in this new, exciting work. His first day on the job, Murray had to find a desk for himself. Perhaps symbolically, all he could find was a beaten-up army surplus item in a back storage room. It tipped over forlornly on its three good legs. The new PR director spent the rest of that day in the maintenance shop making the fourth leg.

Public Relations Defined

The first annual report for STPM (October 1949) spoke genially of the School's reputation as a "humanitarian, scientific, and missionary enterprise" for CME. Wide publicity was given STPM through newspapers in nearby cities. A special, popular exhibit of plastic embedded specimens (insects, mammals, shells, human brain sections, embryos, etc.) toured many libraries, including forty branches of the Los Angeles Public Library.

Milton Murray formulated a still broader plan whereby the work of STPM would be brought to the attention of philanthropic agencies and wealthy individuals. With this beginning, Murray went on to become known internationally as a PR leader and, indeed, one of the founders of philanthropic fundraising.

Yet, for Murray, the path was uphill all of the way, a relentless struggle to create a public relations program for an administration that deemed it largely unnecessary. After eleven years at CME, he concluded that for someone to succeed within the Adventist organization, they would first have to make a success in philanthropy outside of the Church. Until proven elsewhere, the Church leadership would never take this kind of fundraising seriously. With this belief, Milton Murray left Loma Linda and took a job with G. A. Brakeley Company in Phoenix, Arizona. As he worked with various foundations and institutions, his professional skills increased and became well respected internationally. After this recognition, Murray later worked very successfully for many years in the central administration of the Adventist Church.

Back at Loma Linda, Paul Shakespeare, a retired minister, continued PR work, mainly as an optimistic volunteer. Halstead remembered his "eternal smile" and his ability "to convert the worst disaster to make it look like it was God's answer to prayer." Ultimately, the PR department of STPM demonstrated that it could bring in money. Then it was moved into CME's central administration, leaving the School that gave it birth childless. STPM, and later the School of Public Health, was left to raise itself up by its own bootstraps and obtain funding any way it could.

To Take or Not to Take

In 1967 the new School of Public Health opened up a debate on the stand the Seventh-day Adventist Church had taken regarding the separation of church and state. More specifically, the accepting of government money. In the 1950s the national shortage of public health personnel prompted the government to provide scholarships for United States citizens studying in an accredited School of Public Health. Such funds would certainly increase enrollment at Loma Linda's new school and assure its financial viability. Would using such funds violate Church policy?

This question had a long history. At the General Conference session in 1893–1894 the brethren wrestled with three issues. Should the Church accept Cecil Rhodes' gift of free land in Mashonaland (now Zimbabwe)? Should the Church in the United States utilize the tax exemption offered by the United States government? Was the *Sentinel* (then the Adventist religious liberty journal) right in severely criticizing the government for giving the Catholic Church an alley in Washington, D.C.?

The initial vote was "No" on all counts. "The principle," the *Sentinel* cried, had to be the same "in the wilds of Africa as on the plains of our own fair [land]."

The land offer in Africa set a precedent. It came about this way. In 1893 Elder A. T. Robinson secured an interview with Cecil Rhodes, premier of Cape Colony and head of the British South African Land Company. Although the company had previously announced it would no longer give land grants to churches, Rhodes was pleased with the Adventist plan for establishing a mission among the natives. Therefore, he gave Robinson a sealed letter to take to the administrator in Bulawayo. The Church expected to purchase the property but discovered that Rhodes had granted them "all the land they wanted," free. The 12,000 acres they chose became the site of Solusi Mission, the first one the Adventists operated "among the heathen."

Two General Conference men happened to be in Africa at the time. The General Conference president, O. A. Olsen, noted the position taken by the *Sentinel*. "[They say] this is all wrong .... I have not given this matter much thought. It may be that they are right." The issue, on the other hand, aroused the ire of Stephen Haskell. Whether the brethren had done the right thing or not, he wanted to know if the *Sentinel* article was "of a Christian spirit or not." If such language as was sometimes used in the *Sentinel* were used overseas, "our work would be brought into the greatest straits in a very short time .... It creates a wound that is not easy to heal."

When the issue of the African land grant came to the attention of Ellen White, then in Australia, she deplored the "unkind thrusts and allusions" appearing in Seventh-day Adventist publications. She reminded one and all that God is the one who owns the world and those not resident there should not criticize work being done in faraway places. Why "bind up the means that God would have set free?" She advised approaching men "in wisdom" and "acquainting them with our work." In 1895 the Foreign Mission Board reversed the previous action and opened the way for the building of Solusi Mission.

Finally, a gate had opened. It creaked, just a little.

9

Life Support for Public Health

B y 1967, the School of Public Health could apply for and receive government scholarships without apology. Accepting funds from government sources for student support was not regarded as a grant to the school. With these student aid monies, Loma Linda chose to provide minimum support for many students rather than to use a large amount of support for a few students. Research funds were simply a contract to provide services, the "uncovering of truth through research."

Another element not to be overlooked was the self-sacrificing spirit of the faculty and staff of CME. In 1919 the University of Southern California (USC) closed its medical school for lack of funds. To no avail, distraught students appealed the decision. "How is it," they demanded, "that the College of Medical Evangelists, operated by a small church, can maintain its medical school?"

"The reason is very simple," the USC president replied. "Dr. Magan, president of CME, gets paid less than we have to pay our janitors."

USC's shut-down at this time opened the doors for clinical opportunities for CME students at the large Los Angeles County Hospital. Also, as a good public relations effort, many USC medical students were allowed to finish their training at CME.

CME's willingness to accept reduced wages benefited the institution for several years. In 1967 the SPH faculty began their work on the regular Seventh-day Adventist wage scale. This fact, more than anything else, appealed to and reassured the world-wide Church. The membership also had other evidence of good will. The SPH faculty met lecture appointments at camp meetings, ministerial retreats, and even participated in direct evangelistic campaigns, both at home and overseas. The School also provided cooking schools, coronary risk assessments, and physical fitness testing—much appreciated organized outreach efforts to the Church and general public.

Where Do We Look for Money?

Financing public health education at Loma Linda has never been easy. With tuition the major source of income, fluctuations in enrollment seriously affect CME's ability to balance the budget. Endowment funds, of course, are always valuable for tiding institutions over the lean years. Unfortunately, approval of an endowment fund for the SPH was delayed until the mid-1980s. That procrastination would cost the School much money, as well as millions of dollars lost to the University.

When certain specialties are in short supply, the United States government has the pleasant tendency to subsidize the training of specific persons and disciplines. These traineeships have been tremendously useful to schools of public health, including Loma Linda. Recently, the Peace Corps has also made similar significant contributions to public health education.

Because Loma Linda has always had many foreign students, generating student tuition income for them is an on-going effort. Many of them came from the United States government-sponsored program in Tanzania. USAID (United States Agency for International Development) and WHO (World Health Organization) have both stepped up to the plate in behalf of foreign students desiring education in public health at Loma Linda. By 1984 the SPH had the second highest enrollment of international students of any other United States school of public health.

Even in the best of all worlds, money crunching perforce changes things. More recently, Loma Linda University has been forced to re-evaluate tenure, wages, and other concerns. These measures brought about the establishment of a new wage scale for public health. The accrediting bodies had been looking suspiciously at the School of Public Health. "How is it," they wanted to know, "that your wage scale is the lowest of all the schools of public health in the nation?" "And," they added darkly, "your wages are low even within the range of payment in your own University." (By 1992, the SPH salaries had come within range of other Loma Linda schools, but not until 2004 did the range of SPH wages come within the range of the other schools of public health).

At Loma Linda, distance learning and the "extended degree" substantially increased tuition income to the SPH for a time. Then, as the extended degree market in the United States became more saturated, that tuition income money dried up again. Overseas programs remain more open and needy but were unable to provide tuition at the level of domestic programs. True, services by the SPH to the worldwide Adventist Church earned some subsidies and regular appropriations. Experience, however, made the School reluctant to depend too heavily on these sources. They could be cut off without a moment's warning. (In fact, just such a sudden amputation took place in 1989–1990.)

Beyond tuition and special gifts, two other sources remained. The faculty could sell their services to increase departmental income. Lectures, consultations, and testing could be offered to other organizations. Here, facilities like the Center for Health

Promotion would shine. Individual faculty members and departments, then and now, are urged to help earn their own way by winning new research grants or other types of income generation.

Far and away, however, the "goose that lays the golden egg" lives outside the institution. For instance, some $40 million has come into the SPH through the Adventist Health Studies. The indirect support that National Institute of Health (NIH)research funds generate helps maintain SPH facilities and services, far beyond the direct cost of doing research.

Storming the Gates of Government

Dr. Bruce Halstead had blazed the trail to external research funds beginning in the late 1940s. After two years' effort, however, he had not been able to secure any funding for his personal passion, poisonous tropical fish research. One day, a colleague stopped by. "Why don't you contact a sun lotion company, Bruce, and see if they would help finance our Red Sea expedition?"

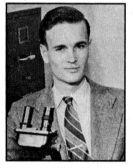

"Um. Good advertising for them and money for us." Halstead saw the point immediately. "Sounds like a great idea. Find me a copy of a sports magazine."

After studying their "text" off the newsstand, they settled on Sun-and-Ski sunscreen lotion. They were mightily surprised when the company showed interest. Sun-and-Ski put up $8,000 for the fish collection expedition to the Red Sea. Later, they financed a short movie in which the divers were shown using their product.

This "commercial" episode, though useful, showed Halstead that significant funding for his projects probably lay with governmental agencies like the NIH and/or the military, not industry. He presented himself in the president's office. "What contacts does CME have in Washington, D.C., or at NIH?"

Bruce W. Halstead helped pioneer externally funded research at Loma Linda. His personal interests were in poisonous tropical fish research.

Taken aback, Dr. Walter Macpherson replied, "None that I know of." He paused. "I suppose research has been considered a luxury that CME cannot afford."

Halstead vigorously contended that if research were given greater priority it would generate more money for teaching. The record tells us, however, that his arguments "did not endear him to many faculty, particularly the clinicians." Halstead knew he would have to go it alone.

On the Doorstep, Cap in Hand

For several months Halstead bantered with government officials by mail and by phone. With NIH in mind, he prepared his first grant application for investigating the bio-toxins of venomous fish in the central and South Pacific. Some questioned whether such toxins even existed, and NIH promptly turned down his application.

Never one to say die, Halstead gathered up his large collection of letters from public health authorities who believed this research to be important. Also, he had completed an extensive review of the literature, something he had begun as a freshman medical student. Early in 1950, he headed off to Washington, D.C. and his initiation into the world of bio-politics. He soon realized that the deciding factor was not the scientific merits of the project. Rather it depended on who was presenting the idea and on the current popularity of the subject matter.

Lacking money to stay in a hotel, he took advantage of the free guest room at Washington Missionary College (now Columbia Union College) in nearby Takoma Park. His first objective was to find the Office of Naval Research. He discovered it housed in a dilapidated "temporary" building from World War I. So much for the status of ONR in the political "food chain." Obviously, successful negotiations needed to begin on a personal basis. So Halstead sought out the head of ONR's biology branch.

Dr. John Field quickly grasped the importance of Halstead's research on the deadly neurotoxins. Hopefully, the Navy would supply the ships, bases, and planes needed. "Re-apply to NIH," Field advised. "I'll refer you directly to Dr. Ernest Allen in the division of research grants and fellowships. Tell them that we will help you logistically with your fishing expeditions, if they will provide laboratory support."

Victory seemed assured. In the process, however, Halstead had to confess several amazing facts to the congenial Allen at NIH. CME had never before had an NIH research grant and the faculty knew little about research. Further, the School of Tropical and Preventive Medicine was a new school that had no money. Finally, Halstead was attempting to plow new ground in a discipline that did not exist! Allen looked at Halstead in disbelief, but listened with a sympathetic ear. He finally asked, "How much do you need?" Halstead responded and was urged to resubmit his previous application.

On June 17, 1950, NIH approved Halstead's grant request for $7,200, while ONR provided $1,140, plus logistical support. On that day the CME's STPM received its first public grant. "Eureka!" Halstead shouted, "we are now in the poisonous fish business."

As far as possible, the state of STPM's research laboratory and equipment at that time needed concealment. The School had inherited the abandoned School of Medicine's South Laboratory. It had been knocked together in 1920 with lumber from an old army barracks. As the STPM renovation went on, Abbott Laboratories (and other pharmaceutical companies) were asked for help in acquiring lab equipment. Abbott Laboratories had an interest in puffer fish poison, and that helped.

Dr. Robert Coghill, director of research, came from Abbott on June 20, 1951, to inspect STPM's research laboratory. What he saw was an empty room (30' x 100'), recently painted green. At one end stood an old lab bench, leaning against the wall and covered by floor linoleum. It was furnished with a few test tubes, beakers, and a Bunsen burner. Also a Waring blender, triple beam balance, and a small table-top centrifuge. And, not to be overlooked, six handmade mouse cages. A freezer stood at the side, containing some poisonous fish Halstead had acquired on the ONR-sponsored South Pacific expedition.

Dr. Coghill stared ahead, shaking his head in disbelief. Halstead broke the silence with the obvious. "You see we urgently need more laboratory equipment."

"What do you need?" the visitor asked.

Halstead fought down the impulse to say, "Everything." Instead, he modestly presented a list of five items (valued at $1,575).

Coghill looked over the request. "I am in favor of the grant," he said, "but I will have to take it to my committee." Perhaps the sheer recklessness of the proposition along with Halstead's ambition appealed to him. In any case, five weeks later, Abbott Laboratories sent STPM a check for $1,575.

Thus began the toxicological laboratory for the School of Tropical and Preventive Medicine.

More Fields to Harvest

Halstead decided to follow his previous success with another military contact. Therefore, he presented himself before the commandant of Walter Reed Medical Center. "Our School of Tropical and Preventive Medicine is part of the College of Medical Evangelists," he announced. The officer looked blank. "It is," Halstead hastened on, "one of the largest medical schools in the western United States."

"Never heard of the place," the officer mumbled. (Ironically, ten years later, a CME graduate, Brigadier General Floyd Wergeland, became commandant of Walter Reed Army Medical Center).

"Well, perhaps you should visit CME." Halstead replied evenly. "You might be pleasantly surprised at what you see there."

A few months later, the commandant with an entourage of scientists from the Surgeon General's office did arrive. And they were pleasantly surprised. Especially, they saw that CME had a gold mine in its relation to the Adventist Church with its worldwide medical mission program. Thus, new relationships were established, and several contracts and new pro-

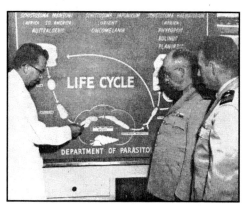

Ed Wagner explains his schistosomiasis research to military officers.

grams evolved, including the funded research of Raymond Ryckman and Edward Wagner. This meeting also helped to initiate the White Coat program. In that enterprise the Army used volunteer noncombatant military subjects (many of them Adventists) for the testing and treatment of various deadly biological disease agents.

After some years, NIH wanted STPM to acquire a pharmacologist and move into a more advanced phase of research. For once, Bruce Halstead's fertile mind had no solution. "My salary is $54.50 a week. Where on earth am I going to find a pharmacologist who will work for that kind of a wage?"

He couldn't. So that attractive project was taken over by the University of Hawaii, which had both the staff and the funding to carry through.

In desperation, Halstead started canvassing scores of private foundations using a striking menu of new approaches. No success. Then, one day, he told himself, "Bruce, you've got to be more positive. Stop talking about all the diseases these marine bio-toxins can cure."

It turned out that the military was interested in hearing about all of the people who could be killed by these deadly poisons. Sadly, Halstead concluded, "If you can demonstrate a technique to wipe out millions of people, there's no limit to the amount of money available."

Calling in the Troops

The Army Chemical Corps received information that STPM, at the College of Medical Evangelists, was working with marine fish poisons that were 10,000 times more toxic than sodium cyanide. "I told them," Halstead said, "that I knew where I could obtain pure tetrodotoxin (from puffer fish)—in Japan." Few people in the United States had heard of this most powerful of poisons. Early in 1952, top brass from the Army Chemical Corps came to visit Loma Linda.

All systems go! STPM would collect the fish, the Shell Company and Cutter Pharmaceuticals would do the chemistry and toxicology studies. In time, the initial STPM grant for $16,480 increased by hundreds of thousands of dollars as CME took over the Shell and Cutter contracts with the Army. At the same time, the STPM laboratories blossomed forth gloriously with excellent new equipment.

Participating in military logistics did add some spice to Halstead's regular work in toxicology. As one in quest for the Holy Grail, he corresponded with Dr. Akira Yokoo of the University of Okayama in southern Japan. This man had reduced the puffer fish poison to its purest form, the first to do so. The Army was more than a little interested in having it.

Halstead stated his terms. "You'll need to give me temporary orders to travel to Japan, at the rank of brigadier general." The rank would give enough clout for him to make this high-priority trip efficiently. In the early 1950s, of course, Japan was still in post-war shambles.

On a military air transport plane, he landed at a United States marine base in southern Japan. There he commandeered a small plane (with a Marine pilot) to fly to Okayama. They landed on a playing field near the university, after it had been cleared of children and animals. Dr. Yokoo was expecting him. After drinking the obligatory tea, the professor showed Halstead several tiny test tubes containing pure white crystalline tetrodotoxin. They represented a staggering amount of very difficult research work.

Halstead looked around the brilliant scientist's crudely equipped laboratory. He understood far more than Yokoo could know. "I felt sick. We were both scientists and frustrated with the conditions of work over which neither of us had any control." Yokoo, naturally, wished to extend the usual Japanese hospitality, but Halstead apologized for his very short visit. Taking the two precious vials of tetrodotoxin in his hands, he thanked his host profusely. Then he returned to the Marine base. Within forty-eight hours he was back in California.

At this time, Dr. George Nelson, a Loma Linda chemist, became head of the STPM work for the Army Chemical Corps. He was able to replicate Yokoo's work, now on a grand scale. Dr. Nelson supplied some of the crystalline tetrodotoxin to Dr. Robert Woodward, a Harvard chemist who determined its structure. In 1965, Dr. Woodward received the Nobel Prize for his work in chemistry.

The End of the Halstead Era

During his busy ten-year tenure with the STPM, Dr. Bruce Halstead was involved in many fish collection expeditions, primarily sponsored by the military services. He authored fourteen books and contributed to more than 300 other publications. His opus magnum was his monumental five-volume set, *Poisonous and Venomous Marine Animals of the World* (each book more than 1,000 pages). With its multitude of colored plates, the printing of the first three volumes took more than five years and was thought at that time to be the most expensive publishing job ever undertaken by the Government Printing Office. (The last two volumes were printed by the Darwin Press, Princeton University). To be sure, the fish business had propelled CME into the world of externally funded basic research. Also, it helped attract students with research fellowships.

Presently, a serious conflict began to surface. The department of medical zoology was simply becoming too large too fast. The expansion of the poisonous fish research facilities with the attendant military income began to concern the CME administration. Even some of the newer staff members at the STPM worried about the implications of the situation.

In fact, the School was now involved with both biological and chemical warfare agents, all top secret. The administration really didn't know what was going on. Both philosophical and ethical questions kept pushing to the foreground. Increasingly, Halstead and Mozar, the founders of so many good things at STPM, began to disagree severely with one another.

The differences could not be resolved. Halstead resigned his position at STPM in 1958 and founded his own organization, World Life Research Institute, which he continued to operate until his death in 2004.

10

Foreign Missions Emphasis

The importance of training missionaries for foreign fields was inherent in Loma Linda training from the beginning. In 1908, one year after the first graduation at the College of Evangelists, a nurse-medical evangelist, Miss Almeda Kerr, answered the call to work in Buenos Aires, Argentina, South America. She became Loma Linda's first foreign missionary. Before the end of 1910 another twelve graduate nurse-medical evangelists had gone to foreign fields from South America to India, China, and Japan. Ten years later, 50 of the first 370 medical school graduates (up to that time), had gone into foreign service. Moreover, 25 of them—the largest number from any American medical school—had successfully passed the British Medical Boards. This achievement permitted them to practice medicine in any part of the then-global British Empire.

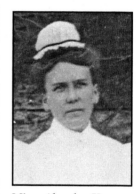

The Impetus for Mission Service

When president Godfrey T. Anderson made his first quadrennial report in 1966, he reported that of the 4,200 doctoral and 2,300 nursing CME graduates, 12 percent had served overseas. Indeed, CME had sent more physicians to world medical missions than from all other United States medical schools combined. This activity indicated that special training was required for foreign mission service. As early as 1913, Seventh-day Adventist

Miss Almeda Kerr, a nurse medical evangelist, became Loma Linda's first foreign missionary as she answered the call in 1908 to work in Buenos Aires, Argentina.

Church administrators were at least saying the right words. "We need a better preparation of workers ... in foreign fields .... [We must pay] special attention to the subject of tropical diseases and tropical hygiene."

At first, this foreign mission training was informal, even haphazard. In 1925, Dr. P. T. Magan spoke of the "custom of the GC Committee" to send a large number of young people to White Memorial Hospital. They were not doctors, but ministers, teachers, and Bible workers, all "under appointment for the darkened lands of earth." Although no one could prepare a course of study for them, they were allowed to hang around the clinics and observe. "We put forth every effort," Magan said, "to make their stay as profitable as possible."

Statistics in 1923 dramatically revealed the need for medical missionaries. At that time, there were an estimated 1,200 missionary physicians in the world, one-third of whom were women; in addition, 500 nurses, 250 native physicians, 200 native nurses and medical assistants worked in 500 mission hospitals and 1,200 dispensaries—small numbers when compared to world needs.

The School of Tropical and Preventive Medicine grew, in part, out of the Adventist Church's need for training missionaries. This would be the first such missionary training venture anywhere in the United States. The first short course was a mixture of health education (to be passed on to the churches) and a knowledge of tropical diseases (to facilitate their prevention and control). The director of the STPM, Harold Mozar, made this his principal interest, and the mission training course functioned more or less continuously between 1946 and 1973. It flexed itself to serve the graduate, undergraduate, and lay-student levels. CME also invited mission appointees from other religious denominations. And they came.

Keep Your Foot Out of Your Mouth

From the start the CME training for overseas missionaries was occasionally criticized. Certain board members looked on the situation with "considerable apprehension." The new laboratories and treatment rooms at Loma Linda, they complained, "far outclass most of our Sanitariums." Should we develop unrealistic expectations in physicians "who must adapt themselves to the meager equipment ... of the mission fields?" In other words, keep the training at the level of a mission hospital.

Still worse things, however, were happening. Dr. W. A. Ruble, superintendent of the Stanborough Park Sanitarium in Watford, Hertfordshire, England, objected to an article in CME's "very interesting and valuable periodical," the *Medical Evangelist*. The writer lambasted the city of Edinburgh for its "idleness ... filth and disease," and for its "slum district" filled with "poor wretches." Ruble had lived there for six months preparing for his British Board examinations and declared that he had never before seen "a more beautiful, more orderly, more inviting city."

The message was writ large. Let not the "Ugly American" (a term not yet coined) display such crass prejudice. "If you cannot say something good about the country in which you are sojourning," Dr. Ruble said, "don't say anything." Let the missionary not start out saying, "This is the way we do it in the States." He added, "This will get you nowhere, unless it be back home again."

Tropical Public Health

In addition to the short orientations already described, the STPM annually offered a pair of two-month classes in parasitology and tropical hygiene—the first such courses ever designed especially for nurses. Along with the usual lab courses and nutrition classes, instruction in nursing and surgical techniques was provided—all modified for tropical climates.

Recommended by the Christian Medical Council, the program attracted many participants, mostly nurses, from other churches. Over a period of 9 years (1951–1960), 74 students from 15 denominations took advantage of the training. Indeed, they had never had such a practical opportunity before. Graduates went on to serve in Africa and Asia, Latin America, and the South Pacific.

At the same time the STPM offered field training for medical students and other health professionals at Boca del Rio on the coast south of Veracruz, Mexico. The School initiated the first course in Mexico in 1949, a summer class that repeated four times over the next five years. CME students immersed themselves in the indigenous culture. They had a rich program with excellent lectures from Mexican professors. Work in local clinics and laboratories. Field trips to remote villages. Launch trips and malaria surveys in the jungles around the Jalapa and Papaloapan Rivers. Institutes and hospitals promoted these activities, and the faculty of the University of Mexico took special interest in potential collaborative research with CME.

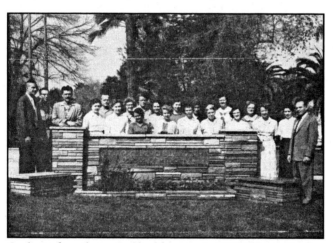

Other spin-offs of this tropical health program included visits to Monterey and the nearby Adventist mission hospital at Montemorelos. To the Ritchie Memorial Hospital in Chiapas and the Autonomous University of Guadalajara. Many distinguished physi-

Graduates from the tropical health course in 1959. This was the first such course ever organized for nurses preparing to work abroad.

66

cians praised this innovative field study plan. "Never before," said Dr. Thomas Parran (former United States Surgeon General), "have American medical students been offered such insights into the problems and needs that exist in other countries." Seventy medical students, along with other health professionals, took part in this mind-and-heart-expanding enterprise.

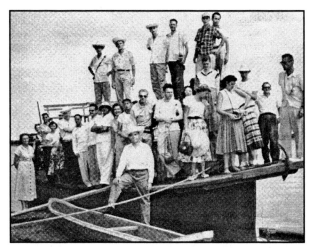

The 1954 tropical medicine study tour of students and physicians, shown here on a boat on the Papaloapan River in Mexico.

These special mission training courses were in addition to the routine teaching that STPM did for the School of Medicine and School of Nursing. In 1961, classes were upgraded to enable students to earn master's degrees through the School of Graduate Studies.

Specific Mission Outreach

In 1964, Dr. P. William Dysinger and anthropologist Dr. John Elick developed a multi-disciplinary proposal for the Adventist Church. They gleaned their ideas from the United States Foreign Service, the Peace Corps, and other mission societies. "This will be a broad program involving several departments," Dr. Mozar told LLU president G. T. Anderson. The need "for a definite, organized orientation" had been felt for a long while.

The proposal called for an intensive eight-week program to convene at Loma Linda once or twice a year. It would help "increase the health, happiness, and efficiency of any missionary, the appointee, and his spouse." (In due course, the eight-week course plan was scaled back to a more workable period of three or four weeks).

This innovative plan of action addressed two urgent necessities. First, rising nationalism demanded

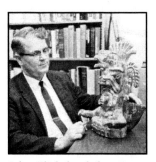

John Elick headed at Loma Linda the first department of anthropology and sociology in Adventist education and assisted the development of an advanced missionary training program at Loma Linda in 1964.

Nine Objectives of Loma Linda's Mission Orientation Training

1. Prepare mission appointee for problems in inter-personal relations overseas.
2. Provide basic instruction for achieving health and well-being (anywhere).
3. Help appointee to foresee and adjust to foreign culture.
4. Present broad view of world political conditions (in a time of independence agitation).
5. Describe various forms of government and international organizations.
6. Provide basic knowledge of linguistics to help in learning any language.
7. Give practical training in first aid, home nursing, and simple treatments.
8. Help wives with homemaking classes, children's Sabbath Schools, Dorcas work, etc.
9. Assist the men to advise the locals on building construction, sanitation, and agriculture.

---

that missionaries must know how to relate to the militant local population and also how to be more efficient in their own work. Second, came the important matter of screening out those people who would always be the square pegs in the round holes.

The misfits needed to be screened out before the Church went to the expense of sending them out and then having to bring them home. In one extreme case, a missionary and his wife docked in a foreign land, made a brief visit on shore, and then refused to disembark. Eventually, they returned home on the same ship. Another man, his family, and his household goods arrived in one of the most advanced island cities in the world to begin their five-year term of service. In less than three months, they insisted on coming home. Sadly, these cases were not a great exception. In 1956 the attrition rate among Adventist mission appointees stood at 24 percent. After 15 years of mission institutes, it fell to three percent.

A Turf War

For ten years Andrews University had wished to have a mission orientation program but lacked the qualified staff to bring it about. Andrews University, in Michigan, was stimulated by the success at Loma Linda and by Loma Linda's 1964 request to the Church for assistance to its newly strengthened program. AU finally conducted its first Institute of World Mission in 1966. At that time the General Conference largely withdrew support from the Loma Linda program. Although president Fighur did recommend that the School of Public Health continue its programs, the General Conference felt obligated to send all its appointees to Andrews. The brethren recommended that Dr. Dysinger assist in the Andrews program. The Michigan institution had chosen a Dutch scholar, Dr. Gottfried Oosterwal, to organize their new program. He held degrees in both anthropology and theology and had several years of mission experience in Indonesia and the Philippines.

On his way to Andrews, Oosterwal spent a month at Loma Linda studying their program, and Dysinger did teach in Andrews' first Institute of World Mission. Inevitably, the LLU mission orientation program began to unravel. With the Church's support to Andrews, the School of Public Health stopped trying to enroll Adventist mission appointees. STPM, however, did have the satisfaction of knowing they had initiated Adventist mission training and had stimulated Andrews to begin its program. Loma Linda continued to serve other denominations, along with the few Adventist appointees who could not get to the Michigan Institute.

To prevent Loma Linda's losing its own mission vision, Dr. Herschel Lamp experimented with a new training format to serve mission appointees. This new course met one evening a week throughout the school year (1970-71) and Robert H. Pierson, then General Conference president, gave the keynote address at the opening session. The end, however, loomed ahead. In the summer of 1973, Dr. Elick conducted the 18th (and last) of the School of Public Health's sponsored programs. The ideal of "a balanced program of mission anthropology and practical health instruction," however, remained. As usual, there had been more non-Adventists in the Loma Linda groups than Adventist appointees.

Nowadays Andrews University sometimes holds their winter institute at Loma Linda—with LLU's assistance. Although the formal "mission orientation institutes" have ceased at Loma Linda, the School of Public Health continues to promote and train for foreign service in many other ways.

11

Tanzania Phase One: Heri Hospital Health Evangelism Training

The College of Medical Evangelists was born in the middle of a "microbiology revolution." In 1905 Robert Koch received the Nobel Prize for his research on tuberculosis and the discovery of the microbes associated with that disease. As a result, health departments appeared everywhere, and improved sanitation helped control infectious and communicable diseases.

By the mid-twentieth century, however, it became apparent that something else was going on. Chronic degenerative ailments like heart-disease, cancer, stroke, hypertension, depression, and diabetes had become the prevalent new killers. Besides, at that time, 80 percent of the world population had no access to scientific medicine. Clearly, good health was more closely related to poverty, politics, and social injustices than to viruses and microbes.

Pioneers of the New Medicine

Three researchers, Maurice King (1966); John Bryant (1969); and David Morley (1973) pioneered the new idea of "integrated development." They established three corollaries:

1. People, living in their own communities, had to take responsibility for their own health.

2. Health does not automatically derive from standard medical care.
3. Health is only one aspect of community development.

These publicized what Jimmy Yen had begun several years before them.

In the 1930s Jimmy Yen lived in a rural county 100 miles south of Beijing. He put together the first practical approach to community-based development. His four-fold program called for: (1) literacy, (2) community organization, (3) livelihood to improve agriculture and income, and (4) health and family planning. When the communists took over China, they found Yen's program much to their liking. Within 30 years "barefoot doctors" emerged and made health care available to one quarter of the world population.

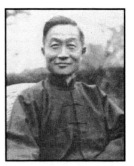

Jimmy Yen, the pioneer of the community based integrated development concept. His initial work was in China, but he ended his career in the Philippines.

The next demonstration of these new ideas is to be found in Narangwal, a village in the Punjab, Northern India. Here Dr. Carl Taylor (b. 1916) pioneered primary health research (1961–1974). Born of medical missionary parents, he returned to India after completing his medical training at Harvard University. Caught up in the violence attending the independence and partition of India in 1947, he and his family worked at relief efforts. When he came to realize that the violence was a symptom of systemic problems, he returned to Harvard for his doctorate in public health.

In 1952 Taylor worked at the Ludhiana Christian Medical College in the Punjab of India where he set a precedent in his field studies at Narangwal. Later, for many years, he chaired the department of international health at Johns Hopkins University. One of his colleagues said, "I know of no one else in the world who has the breadth and depth of experience in international development work as Carl Taylor."

At Narangwal, Taylor trained family health workers ("auxiliaries") to use simple interventions to reduce the main causes of child death: diarrhea, pneumonia, protein-energy malnutrition, and neo-natal tetanus. His researchers actually lived among the

Jimmy Yen's Creed

Go to the People,
Live with the People,
Learn from the People,
Plan with the People,
Work with the People.
Start with what they know,
Build on what they have,
Teach by showing, learn by doing
Not a showcase, but a pattern;
Not piecemeal, but integrated;
Not odds and ends, but a system;
Not to conform, but to transform;
Not relief, but release.

71

The Eight Tasks of Good Primary Care

1. Education about health problems, their prevention and control
2. Promotion of food supply and good nutrition
3. Adequate supply of safe water and sanitation
4. Maternal and child health, plus family planning
5. Immunization against infectious diseases
6. Prevention and control of endemic diseases
7. Proper treatment of common diseases and injuries
8. Provision of essential drugs

people they were studying. Learning went two ways. The villagers picked up outside ideas, and the health workers uncovered simple, affordable solutions to community problems.

Dr. Taylor's findings had global impact, beginning with the first World Conference on Primary Health Care in Alma Ata, Soviet Kazakhstan (1978). Taylor co-authored the study papers used there. WHO and UNICEF stepped forward to sustain the new primary health program emphasis voted at Alma Ata. This began a true revolution in health care which continues today.

Enter Loma Linda University

Loma Linda's first experience in overseas community development began in Tanganyika (now Tanzania), not far from Ujiji where Stanley found David Livingstone on November 10, 1871. Dr. Saleem A. Farag made his own discoveries there in 1956. While searching for pharmaceutically active plants in East Africa, he observed that the African Seventh-day Adventist medical mission institutions had little influence on behavior change, even in the closest neighboring homes and communities. Bad news!

Upon his return to Loma Linda, Farag worked with Dr. Mozar in the STPM to establish an "STPM research and assistance program." They planted this pioneering effort at Heri Hospital in western Tanzania. Both church administrators and government medical officers supported this

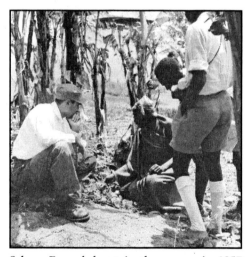

Saleem Farag led out in the surveys in 1957 which prepared the way for the community based STPM research and assistance program in Tanganyika, East Africa.

pilot program where African church workers would be trained in hygiene and the prevention of disease.

The project began with two health surveys. Between June and November, 1957, Farag led two teams to study the health problems of the Waha, the third largest tribe in the country. At 5,200 feet elevation in the highlands above Lake Tanganyika, Heri Hospital sat in the middle of the Waha tribe. Their chief crop was bananas, most of which were brewed into a highly potent beer. Beans and cassava (with occasional beef, fish, or greens) provided the staple menu. Malnutrition prevailed everywhere.

Sadly, Waha housing matched the diet. Thatched beehive huts with dirt floors had one single, small door. People and animals shared the living space, partly for warmth and partly for protection from the leopards. Manure from all sources mingled together in and around the huts. About five percent of the tribe could read and write. Pneumonia, malaria, tuberculosis, and gastroenteritis (diarrhea) accounted for most of the deaths. Sixty-one percent of hospital patients were infected with parasites.

The Model Village

The building started in 1960 under the leadership of the first Loma Linda representatives, Karl Fischer and his wife. Work began by clearing building sites and building shops for tools and brick-making. As far as possible, locally obtainable construction materials were used. Heavy rains often brought transportation to a standstill. The builders became masters of "make do." They had few, if any, precedents to follow.

In January 1962, students began to arrive with their families. They came from all parts of Uganda, Kenya, and Tanganyika. They found ten simple new homes, each with its own separate kitchen-storage area and a pit latrine, plus a community bathhouse. A duplex staff house served the field station director and visiting teachers. The separate classroom, with adjoining laboratory and storage area was built down near the hospital. The total capital investment was only $10,000. LLU sent the director/teacher and provided student stipends and general operating costs, approximately $5,000 per year. The South African Division of Seventh-day Adventist provided the students with transportation to and from the training site. An altogether admirable low-cost operation.

This little African complex must always be honored for being the first community health development project in the Seventh-day Adventist Church. Research and primary health care had not yet become a real movement in the world, and the Heri project was at least 20 years ahead of its time.

Flexing the Curriculum

Traditionally, when workers go for new training, they have problems with their long-term employment. Fortunately, the Heri project would bypass this difficulty. The students entering the Heri program were regular church employees, ministers, teachers, or health workers. After one year at Heri, they returned to their previous

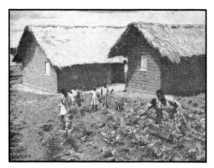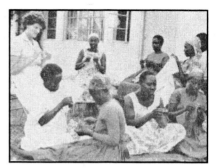

The health training at Heri Hospital was a practical training which included the entire family. Here (left) students are shown working in the home garden and on the right, practicing sewing.

employment armed with additional skills. Their direct supervisors, however, had little background or experience in community health. The graduates needed help and encouragement in applying their new knowledge to their immediate work situations, and were able to receive little such help.

The school program extended over ten months and included both classroom and practical learning. Though coming from diverse tribal, educational, and occupational backgrounds, the students created a functioning village society for themselves. They operated their own duka (general store) and shared responsibilities—re-thatching roofs, maintaining the community bathhouse, controlling vermin, and gardening. Dr. Dysinger's wife, Yvonne, and his mother, Mary Dysinger, guided the women in various home-making activities. They made their own patterns and sewed many garments, by hand. Often they had to take them apart and sew them back together two or three times in order to meet the standard.

The list of those who participated in the Heri project constitutes an honor roll of true missionary enterprise. In addition to Farag, the Fischers, and the Dysingers, there was Drs. Jack Zwemer, Lester H. Lonergan, Naomi Pitman, Tracy Comstock, Molleurus Couperus, Kenneth McElmurry, the Charles Stafford family, and the Reuben Lorensens.

The Virtues of Follow-up

No enterprise is stronger than the quality of its follow-up activity. In June 1963, Dysinger (the field station director), Jack Zwemer, and Mary Dysinger made an 1,800-mile evaluation tour around Lake Victoria. They wanted to see how the first Heri graduates were doing six months after they had returned to their eight different home fields. Their findings boosted everyone's spirits. The students' personal family health had improved, and their enthusiasm for practicing and teaching good health principles had not diminished. The community appeared eager to learn the Heri way of life. Moreover, the graduates had devised several innovative ways to put their new skills to work and were well respected in their communities. Wives, also, were taking on important responsibilities in church and community.

On this happy note, at the end of 1963, the Heri health education pilot project was taken over by the Southern Africa Division of Seventh-day Adventist as a regular program, with LLU continuing to serve in an advisory capacity. Although the concept was as old as the Adventist Church itself, the public health personnel from Loma Linda had pushed this far-sighted plan to the point where it influenced Church leaders in many lands.

In 1970 the Adventist Seminary of Health Evangelism (that is, the Heri project) underwent a detailed evaluation. Findings differed little from the first evaluation. The graduates were engaged in an amazing amount of health education activity despite their limited educational background. They "knew their place" and never tried to "practice medicine" themselves. Most of them established a relationship with a local physician to whom they referred seriously ill patients. The unfortunate disconnect between the graduates and their supervisors, however, showed up. The supervisors appeared to be remarkably ignorant of what the graduates were doing. There was little evidence of the integration of health into the regular mission work. Disinterest and lack of direction in supervision of graduates seemed clearly the greatest weakness of the program. Unhappily, a real marriage between the regular mission work of the Church and health education had not occurred.

In both 1965 and 1968, faculty from Loma Linda led out in two Church sponsored health institutes, designed to serve as refresher courses for the graduates (1965, 1968). Some 130 finished this program and received certificates from Loma Linda as "health education assistants." The flip-side of the educational experience occurred when at least six graduate students from the School of Public Health at LLU took all or part of their field practicum in the community health project at Heri Hospital.

Even with its weaknesses, the project did have international influence. Heri Hospital in the early 1960s was under the jurisdiction of the district medical officer, Dr. E. Tarimo. Much impressed, he said, "The nation needs more practical health educators such as those trained at Heri Hospital." Later, he became the preventive medicine director in the Tanzania Ministry of Health, on hand when Loma Linda's contract with the government of Tanzania began in 1974. Still later the World Health Organization chose Dr. Tarimo to serve as its influential assistant director general. At that time, this friend of Loma Linda was the most highly placed African officer in that powerful international organization.

Arusha Adventist Seminary

Hot plans were a-foot for the first ministerial training school in northern Tanzania by 1974. The Union officers decided that this new two-year seminary curriculum could be strengthened if they blended the Heri program with it. An ad hoc committee convened in Mwanza. They set about detailing a two-year curriculum that integrated health and theology. The Union administrators endorsed this new program. Might it be that the marriage of theology and health would be consummated after all?

Certainly, the objectives for the combined theology-and-health ministry looked magnificent on paper. Then disaster struck. Two of the chief officers accepted calls to go elsewhere. They had been directly involved in the planning and had been expected to implement the curriculum. New teachers came in who had had no part in creating the innovative curriculum. Be it said to their credit, they did seek to follow the blueprint quite closely in 1975–1976. As time passed, however, the distinctive vision of health evangelism at the Seminary faded. Indeed, one could scarcely recognize it as a descendent of the original curriculum formulated at Mwanza. The balance tipped in favor of traditional theology.

So this opportunity to test the exciting concept of integrating theology and health failed. The School of Public Health, as it were, held a wake for the death of that dream. Nonetheless, the pioneers had some satisfaction. The Heri idea indeed proved to be the forerunner of many other health education programs all over the earth.

12

Tanzania Phase Two: Maternal and Child Health

In 1973, the United States Agency for International Development (USAID) announced that the Tanzanian government was beginning a large national effort to improve rural health services. The United States government had committed to supporting the maternal-and-child health (MCH) program. The plans included the building of 18 MCH schools to train MCH aides in the 18 different regions (equivalent to states or provinces) of the country. Moreover, they would assist the MCH policy and infrastructure development for the entire nation. USAID would foot the bill—with one proviso. An American university would have to provide an experienced public health physician on a contract basis. Would Loma Linda University be interested? The answer was a resounding "yes," but who would be the "experienced public health physician?"

History Repeats Itself

A recent Loma Linda graduate, Dr. Elmar Sakala, seemed a clear pick as Loma Linda's public health advisor for Tanzania. He was completing his MPH, in addition to his MD degree, and had committed to specialty training in MCH. Previously he had worked as a high school teacher—another asset. With this in mind, Loma Linda submitted to USAID its letter of interest. The mills of the (bureaucratic) gods ground too slowly, however. Unable to obtain any response from USAID, Sakala had to get on with his specialty training in obstetrics and gynecology and became unavailable to the proposed contract.

Then, suddenly, after months of silence, in April 1974, USAID announced that they were ready to entertain a proposal bid from Loma Linda. They well knew that LLU had already had much experience in Tanzania through the Heri project. But now where would Loma Linda find a specific physician suited to the task?

At this time, Dr. Dysinger was flying the "red-eye special" home to California from the east coast. He had just become convinced during visits to USAID in Washington that Richard Hart could be LLU's technical consultant for this job. Hart, however, was doing his DrPH research for Johns Hopkins University and living at the Kilimanjaro Christian Medical Center in Moshi, Tanzania. The USAID proposal was due in 12 days.

All the way across the country, Dysinger wrestled with a complicated problem. In the absence of telephone connections, how could he formulate a cable and ask the difficult questions about the assignment. Hart, of course, knew nothing of the matter. How would they get a reply from him in time to know whether they could include him in the MCH proposal?

The next afternoon the School of Health administrators would meet for a final decision. That morning, Dysinger received a letter from Richard Hart. It answered every question that needed to be considered. Somehow, he knew all of the details. Whereas Hart had been previously reluctant to commit to work at Loma Linda, he announced that he was now willing to commit two years to be field director of the Tanzania project if Loma Linda was interested. Loma Linda could now submit a convincing proposal.

Dysinger bowed his head, eyes full of tears. God had answered before the request had even been made. Another thing caught his eye. Hart's letter had been posted from Moshi two weeks earlier. Shades of 1905 when John Burden needed that $5,000 for the second payment on the "Hill Beautiful!" Working night and day, Dysinger and the School staff completed their proposal. It won out against the proposals of two other universities.

Just how did this communication providence occur? Mr. Jake Harshbarger, USAID's health director in Tanzania, had traveled from Dar es Salaam up to Moshi two weeks earlier. He found Hart on Friday afternoon changing the oil in his old VW Combi. This man, whom Hart had never seen before, started out: "Both Johns Hopkins and Loma Linda University are submitting proposals for our MCH contract. Both are naming you as their nominee to be the physician-in-charge."

Astonished, Hart had to hear more! After Harshbarger explained all of the details of the project and the appointment, Hart decided in the affirmative, if he could work with Loma Linda. He immediately wrote his acceptance to Dysinger. The really incredible thing turned out to be the fact that Loma Linda had not yet decided to enter the ring. Johns Hopkins never applied at all. Once again, misinformation worked the miracle!

Loma Linda's Largest Contract

Richard Hart's employment at Loma Linda University has, of course, extended far beyond that initial MCH contract. Nonetheless, with his initial help the two-year MCH contract mushroomed into the largest and most successful government project in the University's history. For seven years the Tanzanian project was extended annually, finally ending in June 1981. Evaluation more than ten years later found that this venture had had the greatest sustainability and the largest national impact of any of the many programs that USAID had ever funded. Twenty years later, all MCH aide schools were still operating and mother and child health in Tanzania had greatly improved. Altogether a fine model for many other poor countries.

The background for this project lies in the response of Tanzania's first president, Mwalimu Julius Nyerere. He had set the country on a socialist path in 1967. Early surveys showed that 90 percent of the population lived in rural areas where there was little or no health care. Indeed, Tanzania was listed as one of the 25 poorest countries in the world. Ninety percent of the government health budget went to support a few urban hospitals and physicians. Nyerere set out to "even the playing field." He called for rural medical aides (RMA's) and MCH aides to be prepared to operate in scattered village health posts. These dispensaries would provide primary health care within 10 kilometers of 90 percent of the population.

So the work got under way. Eighteen facilities for teaching the MCH aides had to be constructed and equipped. Also housing for at least 500 students and staff. The 18-month course included six months of supervised field experience. This plan would put a whole new face on public health in Tanzania. More than a dozen physicians and 40 nurses were selected by the Ministry of Health to go for upgrade training in the United States. Eight doctors and 20 nurses in this group came to Loma Linda.

Dr. Hart became the first "chief of party" of the Loma Linda MCH program for primary health care in Tanzania. Many other faculty and staff from Loma Linda University also joined in field leadership, including Drs. Ruth White, Joyce Hopp, and Ezbon Jen. Dr. Dysinger served overall as the project coordinator. Dr. Harvey Heidinger succeeded Hart as chief of party (1976–78) and Dr. P. William Dysinger (1978–1981) closed out the project. Very important to the project were the nurse advisors: Sister Mary Reese, Marilyn Bennett, and Norma Brainard. They came from three different faith communities—Catholic, Adventist, and Baptist. All provided exceptional Loma Linda service to the nation of Tanzania.

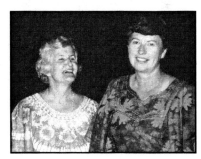

Sister Mary Reese (left), a Maryknoll sister, and Norma Brainard (right), a Baptist public health nurse, were very important and loyal contributors to the Loma Linda MCH project in Tanzania.

Marilyn Bennett nearly lost her life in Tanzania. During a holiday, she was enjoying water skiing in the nearby Indian Ocean. The ski boat's motor quit and a squall blew up in the late afternoon. When the motor finally started, Bennett was no where to be seen. An intensive search began which ended about 12 hours later in the early morning hours when an exhausted Bennett was washed ashore. She recovered well from the acute post-traumatic stress syndrome and was able to complete her service to MCH in Tanzania.

An Assessment of the Rewards

At the beginning of the Tanzania MCH project, USAID asked the Minister of Health if he would object if the contract were given to a church-owned University. After some consideration, the minister decided that he did not. USAID frequently referred to the LLU advisors as "missionaries." To be sure, the term was used in the best possible sense. The workers had extraordinary commitment to their tasks and worked in Tanzania on the Adventist Church-based salary—considerably less than other USAID contractors.

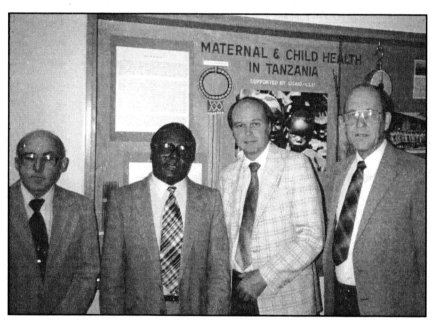

Dr. E. Tarimo is shown here at Loma Linda with the three MCH advisors to the Ministry of Health in Tanzania, R. Hart, H. Heidinger, and P. W. Dysinger. Tarimo was a district medical officer in Kigoma during the Heri health project, was director of preventive services in the MOH when the Loma Linda MCH project began, and later became the assistant director general of the WHO.

Another spin-off came to light. The project required multiple consultant and other staff journeys to Africa. This extensive travel enabled Loma Linda faculty to serve—at very little extra cost—other programs in Africa, Europe, and Asia. Thus the School of Public Health in the Philippines as well as other undertakings in Pakistan, Singapore, and elsewhere came about as a direct result of the Tanzania programs.

Although USAID money was never used for proselytizing new believers, the Adventist Church enjoyed benefits. LLU faculty were always available for free consultation. The Church's mission plane and pilot were frequently subsidized as they helped in inspection visits to the widely scattered MCH aide schools, and the Adventist Church became better known and respected. Loma Linda assistance was also extended to mission groups of other faiths working with health programs in Tanzania.

Loma Linda itself also gleaned good PR credit as it hosted high level government delegations that visited their California campus. Vice president Norman Woods made an official visit to Tanzania. Rarely has any American university had so great an impact on an entire nation as did Loma Linda's MCH work in Tanzania. By the time the Loma Linda contract finished in 1981, Loma Linda had had 25 years of direct affiliations in East Africa. And the Loma Linda concept of primary and community health care had spread around the world.

13

Growing Pains:
Getting Sorted Out

iguring out the relationship between public health and preventive medicine and the medical school at Loma Linda University proved to be a long, difficult process.

A Definition of Modern Public Health

The World Health Organization had long ago declared that a mere absence of disease did not, necessarily, indicate a state of good health. In other words, health is not an isolated factor. It is simply one aspect of a "larger whole," one that must be dealt with in its entirety.

In the early years at Loma Linda, public health and preventive medicine, together, were called "hygiene" and related primarily to the control of infectious diseases. This discipline, however, changed radically during the 20th century. Dr. Dysinger tried to define the intentions of the new Loma Linda School of Public Health in 1966, emphasizing community involvement, the prevention of disease, and the promotion of optimum lifestyle.

The Beginnings (1909–1930)

Since the discipline of preventive medicine evolved slowly in the United States, it comes as no surprise that it followed the same sluggish course at the College of Medical Evangelists, as it did elsewhere. In the first "announcement" in 1909, not a word appeared concerning public health. Dr. Ora Barber, however, taught a small course called "hygiene."

The Basic Tools of Public Health

1. Epidemiology and biostatistics find the causes of disease. Then it inquires as to why some people are susceptible to ailments and others are not.
2. Sanitation, hygiene, and accident prevention try to create the best possible physical environment for health.
3. Good nutrition defines and seeks to provide wholesome food for all. (Not an easy task, considering the increase of world population.)
4. Health education, working within the limits of local social and cultural influences, seeks to influence good choices and motivation in the prevention of all disease.
5. Good public health administration and better medical care organization seeks to control resources and provide services that are equitable and accessible.
6. Mother-and-child health and mental health are other important aspects of modern community health which need to be made readily available to all.
7. International health seeks to use all the tools of public health appropriately in the poorest and most deprived people groups, integrating development principles and concepts (agriculture, income generation, literacy, politics, etc.) with all health programming.

By 1914 the hours of hygiene instruction taught in the department of pathology and bacteriology tripled from 30 to 90. "The subjects of hygiene and sanitation," the college bulletin now urged, "are coming to be recognized as of great importance in the physician's training." George Eugene Tucker and Fred E. Herzer of the department of pathology taught as "special lecturer[s] in preventive medicine." The needs of water systems, sanitary plumbing, and disposal of sewage blended with the more elegant studies in "pathology, bacteriology, and clinical microscopy."

In 1916, the basic course of "hygiene, sanitation, and preventive medicine" took on its new name and continued for the next eleven years. Comprehensively, it took in "food inspection and analysis, determination of the strength of disinfectants, diseases of occupation, vital statistics, military hygiene [World War I was in progress], school and personal hygiene, and a consideration of the epidemiology and prevention of communicable diseases." For the next 40 years, the medical staff of the Los Angeles County Health Department taught most of the public health courses to CME students.

The personal health condition of the CME students came under early scrutiny. A faculty evaluation in 1919 showed that 75 percent of the entire student body needed medical attention during the school year. In fact, nine percent of them became bed patients. Blame centered on "over-eating and lack of exercise." A compulsory new course in "personal hygiene" was required of all the freshmen and continued in the curriculum until 1935. Under the guidance of several professors (Donaldson, Herzer, Campbell, and Crooks) the students were urged to preserve their own health.

Early Stalwarts

In 1925, Fred E. Herzer (CME, 1914) returned from a three-year leave of absence in the Philippines where he worked in public health. As the first professor and chair of public health, he taught hygiene and public health at the White Memorial Hospital in the Los Angeles division of CME. Here, students began to get a firsthand working knowledge of practical preventive medicine in a plan called the "Sanitary Survey of a Town."

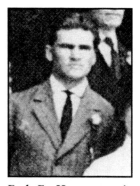

Fred E. Herzer was in the first class of CME physicians and became, after experience with the United States Public Health Service in the Philippines, the first professor of public health at Loma Linda.

Wilton Lee Halverson (CME, 1929) became the best known and longest-serving professor of preventive medicine. He became the first CME graduate to earn the doctor of public health degree (Yale University). During his 31 years of part-time teaching at his alma mater, he held a variety of full-time concurrent public health leadership positions within the city, county, and state administrations in California. In 1955 President Eisenhower appointed him to the International Cooperation Administration (predecessor of USAID). Loma Linda honored its own by naming Halverson Alumnus of the Year (1947). Today the Halverson Award is given annually to a student in the School of Public Health.

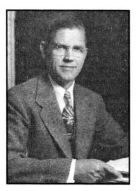

Wilton L. Halverson was the longest-serving professor of preventive medicine at Loma Linda. His 31 years of service to Loma Linda was provided while he served as a city health director in Pasadena, then as long-term health director in Los Angeles County, and later as California state health officer and finally as a pioneer in what became USAID.

A major reorganization of the School of Medicine in 1934 divided the School of Medicine into six sections. In the area of "medicine," public health found a home. Twenty years later, another "housecleaning" in the School of Medicine produced the department of preventive medicine and public health. Dr. Harold Mozar became the first full-time faculty member to be given this responsibility. Was the old "sanitarium idea" about to find a place to stand in the sun after all? Maybe.

Having carefully studied all available models, Mozar set out to make the curriculum more prevention and community oriented. In the second year, the medical students picked up the principles of epidemiology and statistics. Dr. Robert Woods, CME's first statistician, provided the latter course-component. Health education and promotion occupied the third year.

In the summer, sandwiched between the third and fourth years, medical students had the choice of one of three electives: (1) research, (2) a one-month general practice preceptorship, or (3) a one-month tour of Mexico to see public health in a foreign country and to observe environmental problems in the tropics.

Although titles and chair position shuffled around for some time, the School of Public Health began in 1967 with dean Mervyn G. Hardinge. He also served as chair of preventive medicine, within the School of Medicine. In a matter of a few years, however, preventive medicine in the medical school began to struggle up a very slippery slope.

No One in Charge: A Power Failure

Between 1973 and 1987 preventive medicine passed through a debilitating "wilderness experience." The School of Medicine did not list it in its bulletins, and no faculty name was attached to it. Still, someone had to teach preventive medicine and public health to prepare students for the National Board exam. This was quietly arranged, usually by a secretary in the dean's office. Edwin Krick and Raymond West served as consultants, but to all intents and purposes, no one was in charge.

Although not instantaneous, the resurrection of the department of preventive medicine in the School of Medicine did begin in 1986. The Board action re-instituting preventive medicine, however, insisted that "no new monies" would be required and that all parties would find the plan "acceptable."

Partially as a result of the Kellogg-funded Model Preventive Medicine Teaching Centers Workshop, which convened on the Loma Linda campus in 1986, a new emphasis evolved. Instead of the traditional statistics-epidemiology-environment approach to wellness, "health promotion" became the word of the day. Dr. Richard Hart became chair of the renewed department. He stressed the new attitudes that connected with lifestyle and personal choice. Now, hopefully, the LLU public health academic programs would have a very practical orientation.

The School of Medicine *Bulletin* (1989–1991) records the results of serious University financial difficulty and the temporary merger of the SPH into the School of Medicine DPH&PM. This meant that department was responsible for:

1. Teaching of public health and medical students and PM residents,

2. Research (Center for Health Research), and

3. Clinical services (Center for Health Promotion).

·   After that difficult period, the SPH again became an autonomous School with its own programs, but a close relationship with the School of Medicine has been maintained. Preventive medicine at Loma Linda became well recognized as a clinical specialty in contrast to most universities where it is considered a basic science discipline. The Loma Linda preventive medicine medical group is one of the regular practice groups within the School of Medicine. New terms came into use: population based medicine, information sciences, evidence-based medicine, and lifestyle medicine.

The general preventive medicine residency began at Loma Linda in 1979 and has always emphasized a unique combination of preventive medicine with primary care. In 1993 the program was reviewed by the American College of Preventive Medicine and was recognized as one of the ten model programs among the more than 80 preventive medicine residencies in North America.

In 2000, an occupational medicine emphasis was added. In 2003, Richard Hart turned over the chair position of the department of preventive medicine to Wayne S. Dysinger, a physician boarded in both preventive and family medicine. Dysinger began developing and strengthening a new sub-specialty in lifestyle medicine. In 2006 this new specialty was officially recognized and approved by both the American Board of Preventive Medicine and the American Board of Family Medicine, the first program in the world to be thus recognized. Training in lifestyle medicine at Loma Linda began in July 2006 in a residency that is jointly administered by the departments of preventive medicine and family medicine. With its unique history, it is very appropriate that Loma Linda pioneer the new specialty of "lifestyle medicine."

14

A Place to Stand in the Sun?

The 1960s seethed with unrest. While America fought a war in Vietnam; at home, people roved college campuses and city streets protesting that same war. The "flower children" blossomed out of San Francisco.

The Tumultuous '60s

Three separate public health entities had evolved on the Loma Linda campus. Personality conflicts and other problems rendered peace and cooperation in very short supply.

In 1958 Dr. Halstead resigned from CME to form his own research institute. While the future of the School of Tropical and Preventive Medicine was threatened, its service to "mission stations" was reaffirmed. Drs. Harold Mozar and Saleem Farag remained as director and co-director, respectively, of the STPM and its name was changed to division of public health and tropical medicine (DPH&TM)

Dr. Frank Lemon, the university's first epidemiologist, had separated from STPM to work full time in the medical school. There in the department of preventive medicine he had initiated the beginnings of the Adventist Health Study. Meanwhile, the third entity, the School of Nutrition and Dietetics, tottered on the brink of extinction.

Otherwise, on September 10, 1960, the College Church held its last service in Burden Hall, and the members marched across the campus to the new building that was later to be called the University Church. Other significant events included the formation of the Board of Councilors, with Jerry L. Pettis as its first chair (1961). The College of Medical Evangelists became Loma Linda University on July 1, 1961.

In 1963 a continued tug of war ensued over the divided campus—the Los Angeles division and the Loma Linda division. The separation had existed for fifty years. Although most people could see that consolidation would be a good idea, there was little agreement on which way the move should go. Many of the Los Angeles faculty declared that the clinical teaching needs of the medical school could not be met in "rural" Loma Linda. On September 17, 1963, the Board voted the long debated and difficult decision to concentrate all medical school teaching on the Loma Linda campus. Soon after, White Memorial Hospital was transferred to the jurisdiction of the Southern California Conference of Seventh-day Adventists.

Groundbreaking for the new multi-million dollar LLU Hospital occurred in June 1964. It was the largest building the Seventh-day Adventist Church had ever conceived, up to that time. In September 1970 it became the Loma Linda University Medical Center.

Serious Conflicts

Meanwhile, a considerable amount of bad blood had boiled up among the several public health "entities" at Loma Linda. Mighty disagreements arose among the STPM staff and the School of Medicine staff, both housed in the former South Laboratory, known at that time as the STPM Building.

The School of Medicine's department of preventive medicine had its office quarters on the second floor. The division of public health and tropical medicine occupied the rest of the old STPM building on the lower campus. The chair of the Board invited the warring parties to come forward and make their views known. The conflict waxed so hot that a new outside stairway had to be built to the School of Medicine offices upstairs. It served

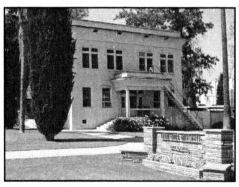

a dual purpose—as a fire escape and as a way for the preventive medicine personnel to have a private entrance.

Although the issues between these two groups had been smoldering for some time, in 1962 real flames erupted. The chairs on either side visited the University president (separately), each recommending that he "do something." Even "if heads had to roll!" At the same time, Dr. Mervyn Hardinge was enjoying tranquility as chair of pharmacology. He was enjoying the considerable amount of external funding for research he had generated.

The newly attached steps to the second floor of the STPM Building. These steps not only served as a fire escape, but also assisted the School of Medicine preventive medicine personnel to enter the building and avoid the STPM staff.

One morning, however, Hardinge lost some of his serenity. "Mervyn, would you join a small ad hoc group in my office tomorrow morning?" President Anderson sounded weary and worn. "We have a complete impasse among the public health programs."

The consensus in the ad hoc group was that a powerful "czar" should be chosen to knock public health heads together, as it were, and force peace upon the warring parties. Hardinge disagreed. "Why not bring them all together in a common goal? Let them all work under the umbrella of a school of public health."

Hardinge went on to outline a potential school of public health staff. The DPM&PH in the medical school, directed by Frank Lemon and Richard Walden, could be the nucleus for an epidemiology department. Mozar and Farag could provide the foundation for a department of health education (and a department of tropical health). The ailing School of Nutrition and Dietetics could become a department of nutrition. In theory, this plan appeared faultless, except for one thing. Lack of money.

Organizing a new University, combining two campuses, building a new Medical Center—all of these expenditures made the Church administrators exceedingly nervous. How could anyone at Loma Linda think of starting yet another school. The turmoil went on for two more years. Occasionally, the ad hoc committee met and tried to relieve the pressure, but they made no progress in resolving the deep-seated conflicts.

Taking a Stand

Exactly what prompted the sudden decision probably will always remain a mystery. On a late Sunday afternoon in May 1964, however, Hardinge received a call from the president. "I want you to prepare a proposal for a Loma Linda University School of Public Health for the Board of Trustees."

Hardinge dusted off his hands. He'd been working quietly at home, doing his yard work. "When do you want it done?"

"Tomorrow morning. Be there at 10 o'clock."

Hardinge drew a long breath. "You haven't given me much time." He eased himself down into a chair by the kitchen table. "But I will do what I can." After a quick shower, he hurried over to his office to work on the proposal. All he could manage was a brief two-page outline. That would simply have to do.

At the Board meeting the next day, the results were nothing short of miraculous. One of the facts of corporate life is that many forests are felled and hours of writing and reading are expended on massive reports and proposals. Full of professional jargon and extended through murky swamps of verbosity, these heavy burdens may cause otherwise intelligent people to quail. Pleased with the precise outline and the hope of settling the campus conflict, board members, almost airily, voted to approve the outline "in principle." Further refinements and budget matters should be presented at the August board meeting, three months hence. Praise be for clear thinking and brevity!

Making the Blueprints

The next day, president Anderson authorized Hardinge to find out what, exactly, would be required to develop an accredited School of Public Health. Hardinge went first to Washington, D.C. to the headquarters of the American Public Health Association. Next he visited the dean of the School of Public Health at Columbia University, New York. Back home in California, he checked out the School of Public Health at UCLA (University of California Los Angeles). Finally, he sat down with Robert Cone, Loma Linda University's vice president for financial affairs, to work out a five-year projected budget.

All was ready for the board on August 25, 1964. As Hardinge carefully read the proposal, a member interrupted. "What's it going to cost?" The eternal question, of course.

"It will cost a lot more than you can imagine." Hardinge wanted to be transparently honest. "The vice president for finance will present the details."

Next, Robert Cone rose to his feet. "As Dr. Hardinge has said, it's going to cost a whale of a lot of money." He barely got into his report when another interruption came.

"I move we establish a School of Public Health," a Board member cried. Euphoria seemed to seize the whole room.

Instantaneously, another interjected, "I second the motion."

Unbelievably, a third voice chimed in, "Question on the motion." The vote to start the new School was unanimous! No real discussion ever took place!

So What Did We Get?

Now everyone had to "cut to the chase," and get on with the project. A new division of public health (DPH) would be implemented within the next six days. On September 1, 1964, Dr. Mervyn Hardinge was named director. The action described itself as "the first step towards a Loma Linda University School of Public Health." Although the projected opening was scheduled for July 1, 1967, Hardinge felt 1969 to be a more realistic goal. Dysinger was dispatched to assure the affiliates in Africa and New Guinea that their future was secure.

This "miracle vote" did not, however, preclude more grief. The naming of Hardinge as the "dean-to-be" was taken as a rebuff by Mozar and Farag. Taking it as a vote of "no confidence," they resigned. In fact, they subversively counseled with the dean of UC School of Public Health at Berkeley, then chair of the SPH accrediting organization. They came up with at least a dozen reasons why LLU was not ready to operate a School of Public Health. Frank Lemon, chair of the medical school portion of the public health puzzle, took a study leave and never returned to the active faculty of LLU.

Under these circumstances, Mervyn Hardinge had cause to wonder whether he ought to be the organizing dean of the new School of Public Health. After all, he had already made several major changes in his professional career. He had first trained for the gospel ministry, then took medicine and post-graduate study in orthopaedic surgery, which led to teaching in anatomy, then had gone to Harvard for his DrPH degree in nutrition. More recently he had gone to Stanford University for his third earned doctorate, a PhD in pharmacology. Besides, things were going so well in the department of pharmacology, why shift gears again?

Together Mervyn and his wife Margaret prayed for guidance. One verse kept coming to their minds: "Commit your ways unto the Lord, and He will direct your paths" (Psalm 37:5). Against the advice of colleagues and many friends, he simply replied, "Lord, if this is what You want me to do, I'll do it. Give me the wisdom I need."

Hardinge had been planning a sabbatical year beginning in the autumn of 1964, but the University administration persuaded him to postpone it for a year. Having given his consent, Hardinge was just leaving the president's office. "Do you really think," Anderson asked, "that you can find a faculty for a School of Public Health". The recent resignations had left some very large cavities.

"If the Lord wants a School of Public Health at Loma Linda," Hardinge replied, "he has a faculty somewhere out there. It is my task to find them."

Amazingly, a number of men and women stepped forward, willing to study in various universities to prepare themselves in the necessary specialty areas. Hardinge had a straight forward method of recruiting faculty. "Firstly, I confirm their spiritual dedication to the mission of the School. Secondly, I confirm their scientific qualifications. Only when they meet both criteria do I offer them a position."

The initial faculty of 25 carried heavy course loads, attended professional meetings, and fulfilled numerous other assignments. They helped organize the Public Health Association of Seventh-day Adventist's (1965). They assisted in the first Seventh-day Adventist live-in lifestyle pilot program in Louisiana (1966). Then came camp meetings, a field school of evangelism, various medical self-help programs, and the founding of a new Loma Linda community services council. And much more besides!

Hardinge spent most of his sabbatical year (1965–66) in studies in Europe and Africa, with stops in India and the Far East, en route home. Dysinger suggested specifically that Hardinge stop over in Hawaii to visit the newly-accredited School of Public Health at the University of Hawaii, Honolulu. The idea had been formulated at the last minute, and Hardinge had no time to make arrangements before he left Japan.

Already experienced, as we have seen, in sudden turns of plans, Hardinge went directly to the University in Hawaii. "May I see the dean?" he asked the accommodating secretary.

"I'm sorry," she replied, "he's in Indonesia."

"How about the associate dean?"

"He's in the United States on vacation," she replied forthrightly. People were entitled to lawful holidays.

Hardinge's options diminished by the minute. "Then, may I speak to a senior faculty member?"

Now the astonishing truth about the fledgling School of Public Health came out. "We don't have any," the secretary admitted. "Just what did you have in mind," she added. "Maybe I can help you."

"Well, at my university we are planning a school of public health. I want to find out exactly what you did to meet the accreditation requirements."

The lady at the desk brightened up immediately. "Oh, you want to see Mrs. Tabochi. She knows all about that."

Indeed, she did. Mrs. Tabochi provided Hardinge with details of their proposal and their budgetary projections. Indeed, this very gracious lady probably knew more than either of the absent men. It was evident that Hawaii had been accredited on the basis of its plans, not its resident faculty.

Dr. Hardinge flew out of Honolulu grateful for the information he had gleaned. He also realized that LLU already had more organization and faculty than the University of Hawaii had. He decided to apply immediately for accreditation. He arrived home to find that Dysinger had already cased out all of the schools of public health in the United States. He had also prepared plans for the curriculum, in consultation with the existing Loma Linda faculty.

With the encouragement of the Loma Linda administration, Hardinge called the APHA (American Public Health Association). "Please schedule a site visiting team to check us out." The groundwork had been thoroughly done, and, in October 1966, the three examiners unanimously recommended Loma Linda for accreditation.

So, was Loma Linda home free, then? Not quite.

Dr. Chuck Smith of UC Berkeley was chair of APHA's accrediting committee. He dragged his feet at the fall meeting and managed to delay the decision until the spring of 1967. A huge, dark cloud of disappointment settled over the campus. With that delay, the University lost a grant of more than $800,000. It would have been viable only if accreditation occurred before November 15. Had Smith been that much influenced by the negative campaign waged by unhappy Loma Linda public health administrators? Maybe.

Then, just before Christmas, Dr. Chuck Smith died of a heart attack. Now the ugly politics of the case came to light. Hardinge learned from Smith's successor that Smith "had a conflict of interest. He did not want another School of Public Health in California to compete with his school."

On February 8, 1967, the Loma Linda University Board officially transformed the division of public health into the University's sixth professional school, the School of Public Health. Hardinge served as the first dean, Richard Walden as assistant dean, and Dysinger as assistant to the dean.

On June 23, 1967, the Loma Linda's School of Public Health received full accreditation, the fifteenth such school in the United States. Teaching under this new status began July 1, 1967. By October the new School was inducted into the fellowship of the Association of Schools of Public Health.

During that summer, another pot was cooking. Loma Linda University and La Sierra College (20 miles distant) were "betrothed" on July 1, 1967. An expensive, unwieldy, and uneasy merger. David J. Bieber replaced Godfrey T. Anderson as president. The following week, on July 9, the new LLU Medical Center admitted its first patient, and 125 other patients transferred in from the old Sanitarium and Hospital up on the old Hill.

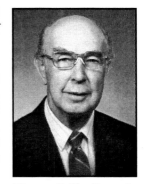

Mervyn G. Hardinge, the first dean of the School of Public Health at Loma Linda, serving as dean from 1967 until 1977.

Finding a Place to Live

The School of Public Health benefited from some of these changes. Deemed as fire hazards, the Annex to the original hotel and the old STPM building (South Laboratory) were demolished. The administration allotted the renovated second Loma Linda Sanitarium and Hospital (now Nichol Hall) to the School of Public Health and the School of Allied Health Professions. One and all busied themselves about settling into their new quarters and enjoying their new honors.

During Hardinge's sabbatical absence, P. William Dysinger had served as acting director. The following year, Dysinger was back to organizing the academic program of the School, and Hardinge took up the general oversight of the organization. Again, he wrestled with the budget and the recruitment of faculty. In the wake of the previous upheaval, the collegiality between these two men was a vast relief to themselves, as well as others.

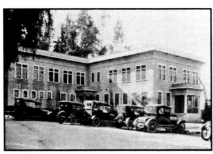

Right: Nichol Hall, the renovated second Loma Linda Sanitarium and Hospital, is now the home of the School of Public Health (and the School of Allied Health Professions).

Left: The original South Hall initially provided laboratory and clinic space for the medical school; later it became the STPM building and provided, later still, the first offices for the School of Public Health.

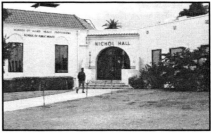

From the beginning of the School, dean Mervyn Hardinge began an exciting period of recruiting faculty and developing new programs. Everyone understood their connection to the sponsoring church organization. As a matter of course, the SPH faculty spent much time lecturing at annual camp meetings, assisting in doctor-minister retreats, and even joining directly in evangelistic efforts in the United States and overseas.

The Academic Programs

Since the 1960s, the School of Public Health has offered an increasingly rich menu of intellectual fare, including the following degrees:

1. Bachelor of science in public health (BS) had first appeared in the SAHP and was revamped in the SPH in 1976 and continued until 1982.
2. Bachelor of science in public health (BSPH) was initiated in 1998 covering three areas: biomedical data management, health geographics, and wellness management.
3. Master of public health (MPH) has always been the "work horse" of the School, the traditional qualifying degree for public health professionals. Flexible enough to combine with degrees in other schools and to cross several disciplines, the MPH (by 2004) offered majors in biostatistics, epidemiology, community wellness, environmental and occupational health, health administration, health education, international/global health, maternal and child health, nutrition, and public health practice.
4. Master of health administration (MHA), a new degree for administrators, began in 1979. (In 2005 this degree was transformed into a new health emphasis MBA in the department of health administration.)
5. Master of science in public health (MSPH) is a research or specialized degree offered at various times by health education, international health, biostatistics and epidemiology, and environmental health. For instance, it was first designed in health education for science teachers, ministers, social workers, and others with the ability to work with behavior change and minister to the whole person (body and spirit). The MSPH degree is also suited to those who seek in-depth specialization in one area of public health.

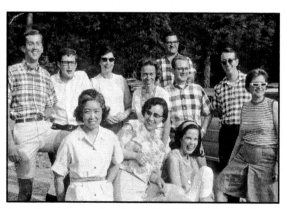

An informal portrait of the first MPH class at Loma Linda in 1967.

6. The master of science degree (MS) is given through the Faculty of Graduate Studies to those who complete requirements in nutrition.

7. The doctor of health science (DHSc), open to those who have "a suitable background in the natural and social sciences," began in 1972. A graduate had opportunities to serve as a health counselor, a lecturer or teacher of health, an administrator of a private or public health agency, an administrator of health promotion (preventive medicine), or an organizer/administrator of community and/or church-health education programs. By 1989, 153 students had graduated from this doctoral program. In 1991 the DHSc was transformed into the preventive care doctor of public health degree program with a requirement for research and a thesis.

8. The doctor of public health (DrPH) degree program began in the Loma Linda department of epidemiology in 1979 and required an original research project and a dissertation. Other DrPH programs were inaugurated in: health education (1981); nutrition (1986) and preventive care (1991); and international health (1995).

Big Brother is Watching

The offering of degrees inevitably draws the careful scrutiny of one or more accrediting bodies. No reputable university, of course, wants its degrees to signify little or nothing beyond the paper on which they are printed. Academic excellence must prevail.

At the start, in 1967, the School of Public Health began with an initial accreditation for two years. It encompassed seven areas: public health practice, biostatistics, epidemiology, environmental health, nutrition, health education, and tropical health. In 1969 an extensive self-study report awaited the site visitors from the Council on Education for Public Health (CEPH) and the School of Public Health received the highest and longest period of accreditation then available. Under Dysinger's tenure as associate dean for academic affairs, a third self-study produced good results in securing accreditation for the maximum possible time of five years. The CEPH visitors admired rather than condemned Loma Linda's church-oriented School of Health—the only one of its kind in the nation.

So far, so good. Accreditation would still figure largely, however, in the difficult days to come.

15

The Woes of
the Neglected Child

Over the years at Loma Linda, public health and medical evangelism have maintained a stout corps of supporters. Unfortunately, on the other side of the aisle, stood those who had no interest or who actively opposed this branch of work at the University.

Success in this kind of academic endeavor depends on two important components. First, administrators must understand the needs of the program and be able to bring resources together at critical times. Second, the university president must fairly represent the faculty and all programs to the Board of Trustees, the legal governing body. How he/she presents a case can greatly influence the subsequent actions of the Board.

Real life sometimes falls far short of this ideal. In the 1970s, the LLU president obtained approval from the Board to hire an architect to prepare a five-year plan for the physical development of the Loma Linda campus. Eventually, the proposal was laid before the Board. Members of the School of Public Health searched to find their assigned location. "Where does the School of Public Health fit in?" they inquired. A sinking feeling of suspicion and dread settled over them. "All of the other schools in the University have a place," they observed.

"We'll find some place for your School at the appropriate time." The administrative reply brooked no argument. The morale of the public health faculty, of course, diminished measurably. In fact, the SPH never was included in this master plan, nor was the matter ever mentioned again.

Not surprisingly, out of this context, rumors frequently circulated about a planned closure of the School of Public Health. Would that be a self-fulfilling prophecy?

Is Anyone in Charge?

Poor communication between faculty and administration at LLU has often been cited in accreditation reports. Both University administration and the Board lacked knowledge and interest in the philosophy and practices of public health. Moreover, when an LLU Board member also chaired the Board of a competing institution, a conflict of interest naturally occurred.

As an invitee to one Board meeting, Dr. Mervyn Hardinge faced this opposition with singular courage. A financial officer from the General Conference persistently criticized the School of Public Health. After one of his tirades, another Board member said, "I would like to hear what dean Hardinge has to say."

Dean Hardinge had a good deal to say. "Members of the Board, I must speak frankly to you this morning. Not one of you knows anything firsthand about the School of Public Health, and that includes the president of the university. Not one of you has ever set foot in the School of Public Health, spoken to any of our administration, or talked with a single member of the faculty."

Hardinge had some very specific charges to make. Board members came to meetings with other agenda items on their minds. After making one of his derogatory speeches, the General Conference treasurer was wont to take half a dozen Union presidents to an adjoining room for a sub-committee. With no idea of the content of the discussion, they would return to vote on whatever motion was up for grabs.

"You, Ladies and Gentlemen," Hardinge said, "make literally life-and-death decisions regarding programs about which you know nothing."

A propos of the point he was making, Hardinge recalled an episode from his own post-graduate studies at Harvard University which illustrated a different attitude. While working one day at his bench in the nutrition laboratory, he was visited by five distinguished gentlemen: the president of the university, the dean of the Harvard SPH, and the chair of the nutrition department. The other two members of the Board of Overseers (Trustees) were the president of the Bank of Boston and the CEO of Banding Corporation.

Urging Hardinge to "tell what's on your heart," the three top Harvard administrators stepped out of the room, leaving the two Board members to question him. For the next fifteen minutes Hardinge answered an enormous range of detailed questions regarding his entire experience at Harvard. Questions such as: Why did you choose Harvard? Are you satisfied with your experience here? Do your teachers evaluate well your assignments? Are the laboratories well supplied and run? How about the library? A similar investigation occurred again in the spring. On these occasions the "Overseers" also questioned faculty, staff, and other concerned parties.

"I had this same, very positive experience at Stanford University," Hardinge concluded. "I appeal to you. Some of you have been on this Loma Linda Board for twenty years. Not once have you taken time to gain a firsthand knowledge of the institution that you govern."

One could wish that this cautionary tale had a happy ending.

Interestingly, at the next Board meeting it was announced that individual members had been appointed to represent the different University schools. Of the five appointed to the School of Public Health, however, only one actually showed up. Two dropped by one time to say, "We're too busy right now to talk with the dean." The remaining two were never heard from at all.

A Serious Downturn

Some ten years later (in October 1976) the stalwart Mervyn Hardinge suffered a near fatal heart attack that forced him into a medical leave of absence. When Hardinge resigned three months later, Dr. James Crawford became dean of the School of Public Health. When he resigned in 1980, Andrew Haynal replaced him—in time to oversee the fourth site visit, self-study, and another five years of accreditation.

An academic version of "musical chairs" continued. James Crawford returned to the deanship in 1983, replacing Haynal. Three years later, he retired and was replaced by Edwin Krick. The same year, another self-study went to the accrediting organization, CEPH (Council on Education for Public Health). This time the accolades were familiar. A pervasive sense of mission and high relevance to the parent Church and University. Strong commitment to practice and service. Successful off-campus programs. Well defined learning objectives. Plus a doctoral program (DHSc) that was on the cutting edge of health promotion and disease prevention. All well and good!

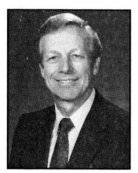
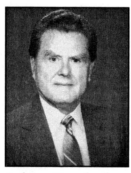
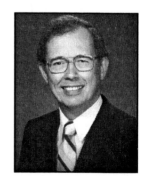

James Crawford, dean, SPH, 1977–1980 and 1983–1986.

Andrew Haynal, dean, SPH, 1980-1983.

Edwin Krick, dean, SPH, 1986–1990.

Now, however, the examiners had found some skeletons in the closet. Why had there been so much organizational turmoil? Three deans in five years must surely demoralize the faculty. Had the SPH failed to focus on traditional public health areas? What about long-range plans for future faculty growth? The School's meager resources bordered on impoverishment. In several vital programs the critical mass of faculty had decreased alarmingly. The salary levels in the School were the lowest of all public schools of health in the nation. Indeed, they were on the low end of LLU's own wage scale. The CEPH called for an interim report in the fall of 1989.

The change of the name to "School of Health" in 1970 had indicated a change of direction. Instead of trying to change government policy, the School would provide a more comprehensive approach, concentrating on lifestyle changes and influencing all people to adopt better health practices. Hoping, perhaps, to lessen misunderstandings and to better fit into the national mold, the Board now changed the name in 1987 back to "School of Public Health." (In this book, the name School of Public Health [SPH] is used throughout the School's history even though it technically was the "School of Health" between 1970 and 1987.)

So now another fearful "force" reared its head, the Western Association of Schools and Colleges (WASC). After inspecting both the Loma Linda and La Sierra campuses, WASC placed the entire University on a two-year probation. It had a long list of complaints, including ineffectual communication between administration and faculty and faulty academic planning. The door now opened to a new "chamber of horrors." Disagreements were evident within a flawed Board of Trustees who had conflicts of interest. There was also concern about low salaries and fundamental doubts about the general financial stability of the University itself. (LLU recognized it could be more than $3 million out of balance for the 1989–1990 year.) To top it all off, CEPH refused to accept the School of Public Health's interim 1989 report. "Submit another report to us in May 1990," they said.

A Year of Trauma

Thus began the most traumatic year for public health at Loma Linda. At the end of the fiscal year of 1989, the SPH showed a $670,000 deficit. Dean Krick told his SPH faculty that most of that red ink came from increased costs in development and recruitment and lack of funding for the Adventist Health Study. He explained to the Board the significance of the unexpected loss of a General Conference subsidy. The requirement to make budgetary projections 18 months in advance made fiscal responsibility a virtual impossibility.

So, in August 1989, the Board wrestled with the mounting deficit in the University generally, and in the Schools of Dentistry, Nursing, and Public Health in particular. A study commission presented the Board with three options relative to public health:

1. Request an annual appropriation of $750,000 from the General Conference,

2. Ask the School of Medicine to help restructure the SPH programs most essential to the Adventist health mission within the School of Medicine, or

3. Close the School and discontinue all academic offerings.

Early in 1990, there was an SPH student enrollment increase, plus an endowment increase of $250,000 in hand. This was not, however, enough to stop the financial hemorrhage. In fact, the operation was in the red for $900,000 in the first seven months of the fiscal year. In the summer, the Board voted for option 2. The School of Public Health would lose its stand-alone status and be restructured as an entity within the School of Medicine.

The local media, as well as the *Loma Linda Observer*, ran with the news: "The Board of Trustees voted by a clear majority to close the twenty-three-year-old School of Public Health." Regrettably, the public report trumpeted the "closure" but took little note of the priority programs (nutrition, health education, and international health) that were scheduled to be born anew, strengthened, and preserved within the School of Medicine.

At the same Board meeting, the Trustees allowed the controversial marriage of the Loma Linda and La Sierra campuses to dissolve in divorce, with La Sierra becoming an independent university. After almost six years administering both institutions, LLU president Norman Woods submitted his resignation.

Amid this upheaval, the Joint Commission on Accreditation of Healthcare Organizations (JCAHO) put the Medical Center and its Community Hospital on probation. In the vernacular: "Get your act together within six months, or lose accreditation." San Bernardino and Riverside newspapers again blazed the dismal tale throughout the Inland Empire of California, even though the long–term accreditation was never seriously in doubt.

Now consternation reigned among students, alumni, and concerned constituents. "Surely the Board acted in ignorance and with too much haste!" The loudest protests came from the alumni who were graduates of both the School of Medicine and the School of Public Health.

Providing for the Needy Child

All of this fancy footwork among the administrators might well leave the average citizen dizzy. Who could wade through such a swamp of detail and sudden change? And with financial and political forces bent on destruction lurking at every turn. Could LLU's School of Public Health actually be snatched from the jaws of death?

The School of Medicine academic dean, Dr. B. Lyn Behrens, met almost daily with the task force and strategic planning committees to grapple with the daunting task of reconstruction. All programs now had to be channeled into the department of public health and preventive medicine of the School of Medicine. Every faculty appointment and his/her salary had to be re-examined. For some, continued employment was questionable.

On April 2, 1990, the Board affirmed its previous action to the effect that the "School of Public Health [should] be restructured as a component of the School of Medicine." Also that its "stand-alone" status would continue through to December 31, 1991 (the end date for CEPH accreditation).

After the termination of the position "dean of the School of Public Health," Dr. George Johnston became acting academic dean of the School of Public Health, reporting directly to dean B. Lyn Behrens of the School of Medicine. A month later, the School of Public Health merged with the department of public health and preventive medicine in the School of Medicine. Meeting in special session, the Board unanimously voted Behrens president of Loma Linda University, replacing Norman Woods. Dr. Richard Hart took up a dual appointment as associate dean for public health and chair of the department of public health and preventive medicine in the School of Medicine.

While all of this was going on, other changes were occurring within the new organization. Reorganization had brought about more efficient uses of financial and faculty resources. In May 1990, a Loma Linda delegation met with CEPH in Florida and was cordially received. A good omen, to be sure. Despite a six percent drop in enrollment, the news was good enough for the Board to vote its commitment by reinstating the SPH as an independent school within the University.

The next visit of the CEPH (December 1991) called for one more year of probation and an interim report from the SPH. The LLU Board was reassured and empowered the University administration to spend $500,000 to strengthen the School of Public Health, especially its departments of health administration and environmental health. After CEPH's approval of the interim report, Hart and his colleagues rejoiced that the SPH again had full accreditation. The 1996 accreditation visit gave the beleaguered SPH another five years of grace.

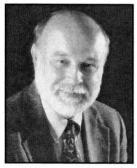 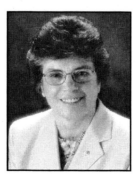 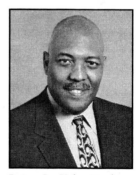

Richard Hart, dean, SPH, 1990-2001 is now (2007) chancellor of the University.

Patricia Johnston, dean, SPH, 2001–2004.

James L. Kyle, II, dean, SPH, 2004–2006.

Just before the 2002-reckoning with CEPH, Dr. Hart became the first chancellor of Loma Linda University and was replaced as dean of the School of Public Health by Patricia Johnston. After her retirement in 2004, she was replaced by James L. Kyle II. This change, however, did not affect the next site visit. CEPH came through with seven years of accreditation—until the end of 2009, the longest period possible.

The story does not end here. Not quite. The child may have been rescued, but a troubled adolescence still lay ahead.

16

Implementing a World View

The long-standing foreign mission emphasis at the College of Medical Evangelists created a natural background for the organization of International Health. From its inception CME defined medical evangelism as the training of (1) foreign medical missionaries, (2) workers for Seventh-day Adventist-operated hospitals ("sanitariums") in the United States, and (3) self-supporting health workers for leadership in their local churches. When the School of Public Health opened in 1967, most of the faculty already saw themselves as "trainers of missionaries." So who needed another department?

The Department of Tropical Health

As it turned out, many important areas of study had been falling through the cracks. In 1968 the department of tropical health emerged. With his long-time interest in affairs in faraway places, Dr. William Dysinger was the choice for the chair position. Fresh from mission service in Africa, Dr. Albert S. Whiting also came aboard to assist in coordinating courses and teaching. The three areas of concentration for tropical health were: (1) tropical medicine (including parasitology); (2) tropical public health; and (3) mission orientation.

By 1970, however, it appeared that the

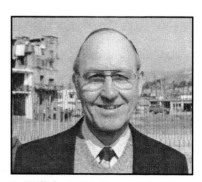

P. William Dysinger, associate dean emeritus, served as associate dean for academic affairs and international health during the first 14 years of the SPH.

department of tropical health had become too exclusive, overshadowing the international interests of other departments. Therefore, the tropical health department underwent dissection and repackaging. Now all foreign service activities were answerable directly to the dean's office. Also, an active international health committee, with representatives from each SPH department, began to function. Since no other School in the University had this orientation, members from other Schools also joined in. Actually, this new umbrella covered a great deal of academic ground for all international programs. Dysinger became associate dean for international health in the School of Public Health, in addition to his work as associate dean for academic affairs.

Picking Up the Pieces

Because tropical diseases are largely the result of unsanitary environments, in the departmental repackaging, tropical health studies came under the jurisdiction of Elmer A. Widmer (a parasitologist) and first chair of environmental health. Dr. Albert Whiting co-chaired the blended department, environmental and tropical health until he took study leave. Then, Dr. Franklin A. Crider took his place. The new department covered a trio of offerings: environmental health, public health parasitology, and tropical medicine. By 1976, however, parasitology was dropped, and tropical medicine began to fade. Collaboration with physicians also waned, until the phrase "tropical health" disappeared entirely from the departmental name (1984).

Now the other elements of tropical health instruction stood at the door of "public health practice," chaired by Dr. Andrew Haynal. Yet another name change now produced the department of health administration (HADM). Maternal/child health and family planning, along with international health administration were transferred in. In short, HADM harbored international health for almost nine years.

Dr. Richard Hart was given administrative control over "international health" in 1979. With the inauguration of the international health MSPH in 1979 came the first Loma Linda off-campus experiment in public health education using languages other than English—Spanish and French. This happened in the Inter-American Division of Seventh-day Adventists (Central America and the Caribbean), with Dr. George E. Johnston as program director. During this time Dysinger was given the first-ever opportunity for a Loma Linda faculty member to be a formal consultant with SAWS (Seventh-day Adventist World Service), now known as ADRA (Adventist Development and Relief Agency). That first outreach to war-torn Lebanon, however, did not succeed.

The years of dancing around the structures of departments had begun to wear thin. It was like trying to find your way home in a town where the street names, house numbers, and landmarks kept changing every other day.

International Health: This One Thing We Do

By 1984, the need for a centralized focus became more than obvious. Dysinger became the first chair of a new department, international health (INTH). Students who were not health professionals had to choose a skill area, in addition to the core department requirements. The rather large skill menu included agriculture, environmental health, health administration, health education, maternal-and-child health, nutrition, and quantitative methods/health planning.

The now-familiar leadership changes continued. When Dysinger took over the preventive medicine residency at the Jerry L. Pettis Memorial Veterans Medical Center, Harvey Heidinger and Richard Hart co-directed INTH. In 1990, Dr. Gordon Buhler, with work experience in India and ADRA International, chaired the INTH department. When Barbara Frye-Anderson, a former Peace Corps volunteer, joined the LLU faculty, she added yet another dimension to INTH. The INTH MPH requirements seemed stabilized in three parts: public health core courses, international health theory and knowledge base, and policy and advocacy issues. When Buhler resigned in 1995, Hart had to step back in as interim chair.

The School of Public Health rode out this transition, however, and in 1996 Dr. Jayakaran S. Job, MD, Dr.PH became the next chair. Originally from India, he had trained and practiced at Vellore Christian Medical College. Four years later Barbara Frye-Anderson was appointed chair of INTH and in 2005 she was replaced by Dr. Ronald Mataya, an OB–Gyn specialist from Malawi who had had several years' experience as senior health advisor in ADRA.

The current roster of SPH offerings gives a good sense of the diversity and scope of modern international health as taught at Loma Linda.

Rotating Modules for International Health (fall, winter, and spring quarters)

1. Primary health care and development
2. Communicable diseases and essential drugs
3. Risk assessment for water safety and sanitation
4. Agricultural sustainability and food security
5. Urban health
6. Traditional practices and beliefs
7. The family under stress
8. Maternal health
9. Family planning
10. Child health and survival
11. Community–based rehabilitation (CBR)
12. Health education and literacy enhancement
13. Complex health emergencies (disasters and refugees)
14. Micro-enterprise and poverty alleviation
15. Advocacy and lobbying

**Six Tracks for the
MPH Degree**

1. Health professionals (100-hour practicum)
2. Non health professionals (400-hour practicum)
3. Peace Corps Internationalist (MPH/MIP)
4. Combination of MD or DDS with MPH
5. Summers-only program
6. Combination with the preventive medicine residency

International health seems at last to have arrived in its effort to address "local issues in local settings as well as in the global arena." Just one more name change had to come. The new title, department of global health stays on course with high purpose: to practice "borderless" thinking, to encourage collaborative partnerships, and to "enhance the quality of life for all people." Since 2000 the student enrollment in international/global health has quadrupled, making it the largest single major in the School of Public Health.

The Capstone Course in International Health

Is it possible that through the decades of shifting sands the SPH at Loma Linda could teach one course annually for more than 24 years? That it would be required of all INTH majors? The astonishing answer is "Yes!" It comes under the heading of "integrated rural development."

Modern international health recognizes health as only one component in the spectrum of "development disciplines." For instance, in developing countries one does not discuss nutrition apart from agriculture. Don't even think of talking about foods that are not locally grown. Also, illiterate people have a hard time getting information. And remember that even road building often directly and indirectly impacts and supports health. Health and all other development disciplines must integrate and blend.

As we have noted, the World Health Organization—almost 60 years ago—defined health as being more than just an absence of disease. Over time one important fact has emerged. Health is much more closely related to poverty, politics, and social inequities than to viruses and microbes. In fact, high-quality medicine in the recent past has been available to about 20 percent of the (affluent) inhabitants of the cities of the world. Doctors and modern hospitals were to be found only there. The largely rural inhabitants had little, if any, contact with modern medicine.

When Dr. Andrew Haynal (CME '48) began a public health tour of duty in Liberia in 1951, he made a practical demonstration of these statistics. From scratch he started a local health department in a rural area. He was assigned a place deep in the bush country some 200 miles from Monrovia. Through both education and agricultural methods, UNESCO helped sustain this integrated health project—one of the first.

At Loma Linda, the SPH leaders had long realized that in order to serve poor communities, the students would have to live and work with the people. Bridging the gap between the World Health Organization and the local Village Health Committee could not be accomplished in the classroom alone. In the summer of 1980, the first integrated rural development field course began in easily accessible Mexico and Guatemala. For three weeks Dr. Robert Ford (of INTH) and Douglas Havens (director of agriculture in the College of Arts and Sciences) led their students through a real "grassroots" experience.

Immediately, close association and group travel were recognized as a "good thing." Especially under difficult conditions, travel is a great test of compatibility and adaptability. After the first heady days of the trip have passed, the realities and rigors of close proximity among faculty and classmates sets in. Managing close association in an underdeveloped country challenges everyone. Students have to deal with local finances and travel arrangements, including the necessities of food and water. Indeed, a multitude of logistical details occupies every waking (and sometimes sleeping) hour for the students.

Integrated Community Development

Recognizing the value of this field experience in integrated community development, the SPH decisively nailed down seven components. The School has provided this course in a wide range of countries in Africa, Southern and Southeast Asia, Latin America, and Eastern Europe. The administrators rotate the field school so as to avoid overtaxing the resources of any single country.

Loma Linda soon discovered that their carefully orchestrated course really put a human face on the problems of international public health. Preparatory to the project, one student researched the causes and proposed solutions to the global public health issue of sex trafficking. In due course, she found herself on the streets of a major city where young men and women were being sold. The

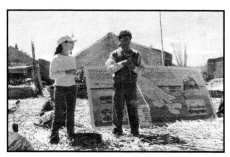

The 2006 integrated development field study was in Bolivia. Here one of the students is shown teaching health on one of the floating islands on Lake Titicaca.

marketers described their "wares" in the most degrading and vulgar terms. The graduate student sat down on the curb, hand in hand with the young prostitutes. As she

---

Requirements for Integrated Community Development

1. A "case study" is made of a region or a nation.
2. The study has to be based in a country with limited resources.
3. Before the fieldwork, the student spends three academic quarters studying the culture and public health issues in the country to be visited.
4. The three-week, on-location course is led by an LLU faculty team.
5. Students meet people from UN organizations, government ministries, and other agencies.
6. Students are encouraged to participate in cultural events and interact with the local people.
7. Finally, students have to pass a comprehensive essay examination to assess their field experience.

---

listened to their stories, her heart almost broke. "Nothing in the classroom or my research," she wrote later, "could have prepared me for what I experienced on the street that evening."

At Loma Linda, time long ago proved that nothing trains one for foreign service better than supervised, personal experience in the field.

17

Taking It to the People Through Education

P eople can voluntarily change their habits and improve their lifestyle through experiences acquired through health education. Then, hopefully, they will be sufficiently motivated to maintain these practices.

Loma Linda's School of Public Health took a unique approach to health education. From the beginnings in 1964, the School recognized that this discipline stood firmly on two legs: the social sciences and the health sciences. Whereas most schools of public health teach only the social sciences, LLU has always insisted on the two, combined under "health promotion and education."

Standing on Both Legs

The social sciences aim to understand people through psychology, sociology, and cultural anthropology. Every society, every sub-culture, has its own modus operandi. Professionals must discover how the population lives, how they organize themselves, and what motivates them toward change. In effect, the community becomes the patient and the public health educator the physician.

The social sciences appeared on the scene of Adventist education rather late. In 1956 Dr. Mozar observed that in Adventist schools there actually were no professionally qualified persons "to teach the social sciences needed for health educators."

Providentially, at the precise moment of necessity, three joined the Loma Linda University faculty. Dr. John Elick, a cultural anthropologist, had been one of the early students in the mission training in the School of Tropical and Preventive Medicine. He chaired LLU's new department of anthropology and sociology, the first of its kind in Adventist education. Then Dr. Betty Stirling (a sociologist), and her husband, Dr. James Stirling (a cultural anthropologist), joined the faculty. All three social scientists contributed much to planning and teaching in the SPH.

In 1980 the health education department added its own behavioral science base which has turned out to be one of the core areas required for accreditation. Dr. Jerry A. Lee and Dr. Helen Hopp-Marshak, both social psychologists and full-time faculty, have further strengthened the curriculum.

The basic health sciences have always had more emphasis at Loma Linda than in most other schools of public health. The SPH has always believed that the ability to know and obey God-given "laws of health" must be based on an understanding of the structure and function of the body. That means the study of physiology, anatomy, biochemistry, and microbiology, in both its gross and micro forms. Basic to life are the more than 600 different types of cells that make up the tissues and organs of the body. The SPH has never apologized for its basic health science entrance pre-requisites.

With its traditional emphasis on the blend of health education and medical evangelism, Loma Linda turned up many sub-specialties of health education. Here are three of these sub-specialties to illustrate how these things work.

School Health

School health programs provide health services in schools (physical exams, vision and hearing training, detection of infectious disease, and first aid). They make health education available to both teachers and students, and encourage the maintenance of a healthful environment (sanitation, ventilation, lighting, etc.). School health programs are usually administered by nurses with specialty training.

Dr. Joyce Wilson-Hopp, a Loma Linda graduate nurse, was the first to hold such a school health position in the Adventist Church. She began her career as director of health education in the Upper Columbia Conference of Seventh-day Adventists. During the next three years, she created health education programs for both schools and churches.

Aware of her Church's need for health educators, she earned her MPH in Harvard's School of Public Health, the first Adventist health educator to obtain this degree. Immediately, the Medical Department of the General Conference of Seventh-day Adventists picked her to develop school health programs for their very large school network in North America. In the course of her nine years at headquarters (1954–1963), Joyce Hopp visited every teacher's

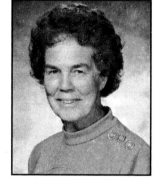

Joyce Hopp had a long, distinguished career in the SPH and the SAHP.

convention, every academy, and many of the elementary schools in the North American Division. Exactly the excellent background for what LLU's School of Public Health needed. In fact, she had already started volunteering at Loma Linda in the early 1960s.

In 1971, in cooperation between the SPH and LLU's School of Nursing, Hopp put together a program for school nurses that led to the California School Nurse Credential. Together with the School of Education, a teaching credential was soon added to the mix. Using the resources of the SPH (1972–1975) Hopp prepared for the North American Division of Seventh-day Adventists the first set of health science textbooks (kindergarten through grade eight). Ten years later, the task was repeated for the next generation of elementary school children. Curriculum guides for HIV/AIDS were also produced.

In due course, her husband, Kenneth Hopp, helpfully moved his law practice to Southern California. Although still busy with two young children, Joyce completed her PhD at the University of Southern California (1974). Highly respected in professional circles, she chaired the health education department at LLU (1979–1983). Her innovative lectures and her editorship of the *California State Journal of Health Education* prepared her way to the day when she was elected chair of the international health committee of the American School Health Association (1981).

Hopp first became an international figure with service in Adventist school health programs in the Philippines with her former student, Marietta Deming. Her early work in the USAID funded project in Tanzania led to several trips to that country where she directed workshops for the teachers of the MCH aides. Although other names might be mentioned, by common consensus it is agreed that Hopp cast the longest shadow of influence over the teaching of school health education at Loma Linda.

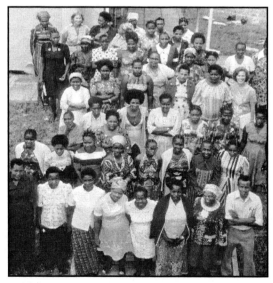

Beginning in the 1970s Harold Googe brought an important addition to school health programs. He and 26 SPH students presented 276 anti-smoking programs to 3,000 children in the Red-

Joyce Hopp (upper right) during a training workshop for the teachers of the MCH aide schools in Tanzania.

lands Unified School District. Apparently no one before had so thoroughly covered an entire school district. President Richard Nixon sent, through his Surgeon General, his congratulations from the White House.

Another interesting exercise involved the Yucaipa Unified School District. What influence might children have in helping their parents stop smoking and thereby reducing coronary heart disease? A large group of SPH and multidisciplinary faculty undertook this unique research. (The findings later appeared in the important text *Perspectives on Community Health Education*). The project documented changes among high-risk parents. As Joyce Hopp reported: "Over half the families indicated that … [the child] was most helpful in making the positive health behavior change." In common speech, the parents quit smoking!

Other involvements kept surfacing. A sixth-grade teacher at Woodrow Wilson Elementary School in South Colton "had no idea that the people from LLU's SPH could be so wonderfully effective in presenting their drug education program." Kim Clark brought his "feeling good program" to the fourth-graders in the Redlands McKinley School. They learned about stress, exercise, and obesity. Then, utilizing peer education, Clark trained 20 high school students to persuade 200 seventh-graders in the Yucaipa Unified School District not to smoke. This activity led to PUFFS (Peers Urging Freedom from Smoking) for smoking cessation among adolescents in other schools. Other school districts benefited from nutritional awareness among elementary students. Subsequently, seventh- and eighth-graders in Redlands and San Bernardino were taught the subject of violence and how to prevent it.

Time marched on, and, after 1999, the general community health education major absorbed the school health program.

Hospital Health Education

Health lectures convened almost every evening in the parlors of early Adventist sanitariums. Dr. John Harvey Kellogg greatly popularized this "parlor activity." Then, as sanitariums evolved into acute-care hospitals, physicians had less time for educating their patients. Eventually, health education could not even be seen to be a function of modern medical centers.

In the 1960s and 1970s, however, a re-awakening of the "sanitarium idea" occurred. Loma Linda had considerable influence in the movement. LLU graduates served as hospital health educators throughout the United States. This discipline has three distinct functions: community education, patient education, and in-service (staff) education.

Shortly after the Loma Linda University Medical Center opened, it hired its first health educator, Joyce Lim, a recent SPH graduate (1969). The department soon grew to employ four persons. Heavy emphasis now had to fall on public relations. People already had a negative attitude about costly hospitals, those "disease palaces" that cared only about the money sick patients paid. To neutralize this situation, Loma Linda promoted major community service programs: smoking cessation, nutrition, physical fitness, stress management, and birthing/parenting classes were some of these.

Dr. Christine Gerken-Neish pioneered, for example, patient education in COPD (chronic obstructive pulmonary disease) and emphysema. The guidelines she developed have been published and are used nationwide by pulmonary rehabilitation programs.

Popular opinion holds that all physicians and nurses are health educators. Not so. Because few of them have had any educational training, in-service had to step into the void. First comes general health education followed by important specifics in such areas as rehabilitation from heart attacks and strokes, cancer management, and diabetes control and prevention of complications. A sense of security is created for both the patients and the public.

Unfortunately, experience has shown that when hospitals face financial difficulties, the first thing they drop is health education. The economic situation worsened, and by the 1970s relatively few health education specialists remained as hospital employees. On the other hand, more and more new hospital specialists today come trained in health education—something not necessarily true in the past.

Corporate Wellness/Fitness Programs

Loma Linda's corporate wellness programs began on the October day in 1963 when Dr. Richard T. Walden announced a new service, executive health physicals. Top drawer executives had finally begun to realize their vulnerability to heart disease, cancer, diabetes, and other curses of Western civilization. Indeed, this check-up would be good for all workers. Everyone needed to know about coronary prevention, stress management, dependency programs, smoking cessation, and other good things that went into a comprehensive "wellness program." Since 1983, all of these elements have been housed in the Center for Health Promotion.

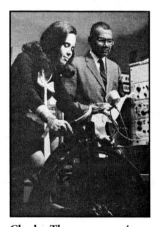

Charles Thomas (born in India) joined the department of health education in 1967. His professional background was in physical therapy and his doctorate in education. Having an unusual flair for promotion, he carried family fitness programs to schools and churches far and wide. In addition to his service on the "Hill Beautiful," Thomas had global influence. Loma Linda became the first university to ever make physical fitness testing available to all students and faculty. At about the same time, Dr. Kenneth Cooper was working on his aerobic exercise ideas. He made multiple visits to Loma Linda and LLU students used his aerobic center in Dallas, Texas, as a site for field practicums.

Charles Thomas overseeing a physical fitness test of a Loma Linda public health student, Eunice Hankins.

Helen Register and others from HLED (health education/department) championed weight management. With good results, they took the "Better Weigh" program to the campus, the town, and local Native American reservations.

In the late 1980s, Dr. David C. Nieman, took over the fitness program and created "Summer Slim" and "Fitnessize." The latter provided exercise "to music in a Christian atmosphere." Nieman took particular delight in testing people like Mavis Lindgren, who held the world title for people her age in marathons. (See chapter 6.) Nieman directed the first studies showing that exercise to exhaustion is detrimental to the immune system. His textbook *The Sports Medicine Fitness Course* (1986), grew out of the fitness instructor workshop and certification program he launched at Loma Linda.

In 1985 the area of corporate wellness emerged in HLED, to be supplanted by community wellness in the 1990s. It served the person who wished to focus on a specific situation in business, industry, or the private sector. By 1998, the bachelor of science in public health took in "wellness management," a move that enabled graduates to find employment in health-related fields or to continue on to a graduate degree.

HLED students always have opportunities to involve themselves in church sponsored programs, like the SACH clinics and SIMS projects. Each one has the potential of tailoring his field work to his personal area of interest. Applied research has always been an important adjunct to health education in the SPH at Loma Linda.

So Who Is Going to Pay for This?

Health education has always had a problem getting paid for its services. Although, supposedly, it is as important as medical care, it is not at the core of disease treatment. As finances for hospitals and other medical care become strained, health education is usually the first casualty. Unreasonably, many consider it a luxury that cannot be afforded.

To establish "legitimacy," a certification for the profession of health education is at least one solution that may prepare the way for such professionals to be reimbursed. The LLU School of Public Health education department has worked earnestly to this end. After long effort, CHES (certified health education specialist) was born. Today, public health agencies and other organizations seeking health educators require this certification. Faculty and alumni from HLED have served on the national CHES board and have conducted workshops. Loma Linda's HLED majors must all earn their CHES.

Today, interest in lifestyle medicine now stands in the foreground of informed public thinking. High risk conditions like smoking, stress, lack of exercise, overeating, and all the rest, are finally beginning to be understood. Health education's challenge, then, is to show that human behavior can change and that disease mortality can decrease.

18

Taking It to the People Through the Church

U nfortunately, the next phase of the health education story is told too quickly. Discussing the attempt to merge health and religion education, J. G. Smoot of Andrews University stated to R. E. Cleveland of LLU: "Sometimes it takes a great deal of effort for an idea to be born." To that piece of wisdom we must add another truth: "And the maintenance of the idea afterwards is seldom easy."

CME/LLU conscientiously attempted to serve its sponsoring Church from the first day of classes in 1906. Although the ideal of medical evangelism waxed and waned through the years, the original vision was never lost. In 1947 the School of Tropical and Preventive Medicine's first effort was to teach a six-week course "in health evangelism (that is, medical evangelism) and tropical hygiene to mission appointees, Bible instructors, minister, and other educators seeking knowledge of basic health principles. The Adventist Church provided an annual subsidy to CME to encourage this kind of Church health education.

As dean of the new School of Public Health and chair of HLED, Dr. Mervyn Hardinge vigorously supported the church as an important site for health education. Today, interest in "religion and health" and "faith-based initiatives" is high. Loma Linda's concept was at least 30 years ahead of its time. Back in 1968, however, SPH faculty were featured at camp meetings all over the United States. A surprisingly large number of ministers came forward to join this new component to their ministry.

Off to a Fast Start

P. T. Magan's dream back in 1938 now appeared to be on the brink of fulfillment. He had said that a minister "of the right stamp" needed to be found, in order to unite medical ministry and the work of "preaching the gospel." Wilbur K. Nelson appeared to be that man. As a member of the HLED faculty, he taught courses in religion and health and planned the congruent training programs. As an ordained Adventist minister, Nelson had had several years of mission service in the Far East, had completed a doctorate in Asian studies, and taken an MPH at Berkeley. From his studies, he felt that ministers, as opinion leaders, could readily adapt to community health education work with minimal guidance from public health agencies.

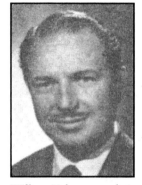

In Nelson's first year as chair of the department of health education (1969), he brought Church health education to a new level. The next year something quite remarkable occurred. Andrews University sponsored two field schools of evangelism, one in Savannah, Georgia, the other in eastern Pennsylvania. On both of these occasions, students from Loma Linda and Andrews, along with health professionals, all came together in a common cause. At this point, perhaps, the possibility of renewing the previously broken "engagement" between the two universities came into the minds of some people.

Wilbur Nelson, as chair of health education, helped to renew the vision of health evangelism in "Better Living" efforts as an outreach of the Adventist Church.

Meanwhile, Nelson, along with Dr. and Mrs. Lester Lonergan and Robert Spangler (of the General Conference Ministerial Association) carried the new "training combo" to the Philippines, followed by Taiwan and Hong Kong. In the same year, Charles Thomas lectured in many Church institutions and conducted physical fitness testing throughout India, Ceylon, Singapore, and the Philippines. The world-wide Church could not help but appreciate these services, especially since Nelson and his assistants prepared a wide range of health education materials for ministers. They also

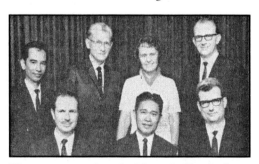

The team approach to health evangelism is shown here by this team which includes Wilbur Nelson, Dr. and Mrs. L. H. Lonergan, and Robert Spangler and other important helpers. They conducted a very successful training effort in Manila, Philippines in 1970.

published articles in both secular and religious journals describing this new ministry of "health evangelism."

Another Courtship?

Another experienced, hard-working minister, Leo Van Dolson, joined the faculty, followed by Daniel Skoretz. Interest in church health education soared. It turned out that more than twenty students at Andrews University wished to take additional study at LLU. Loma Linda's Board asked the General Conference to approve HLED offering its MSPH or MPH with a concentration in religion and health. That meant that it needed to become a legitimate part of theological education.

Perhaps now was the time to try, again, to see if an academic marriage could be arranged with Andrews University. While there was no great enthusiasm in Michigan, an agreement was reached on a conjoint degree that combined the MSPH with the MDiv degree. The theology program required nine quarters and the MSPH called for four. A compromise permitted both programs to be finished in eleven quarters. Many theology students showed much interest in the new approach, and the field schools continued to flourish.

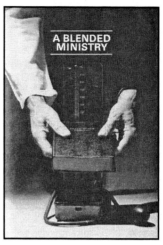

The ideal of health evangelism is to combine the gospel ministry with the work of health professionals, here symbolized by the Bible over the sphygmomanometer.

In 1976, another faculty member, Reuben Hubbard, cheerfully reported that the "health and religion" program had aroused "a great deal of interest beyond Loma Linda" and was headed into a "bright future." At the time, 45 ministers from eleven countries and fourteen states in the United States were enrolled. Hubbard's optimism, however, would ultimately be sabotaged.

While James M. Crawford was dean of the School of Public Health at Loma Linda in 1980, he received a letter from the provost at Andrews University. It began mildly enough, affirming that the conjoint theology/health program between the two universities had "been helpful to a group of our students." Then, came the death blow: "It would be as well to discontinue the experiment at this time."

Dean Crawford did not take the news passively. Knowing him to have been a supporter of the conjoint venture, he appealed to Thomas Blincoe, dean of Andrews' Theological Seminary: "Let's not give up on this, Tom. Somehow God would have our ministers trained in the basic understanding of health ministry. They constantly deal with human beings—body, mind, and spirit. We must find an appropriate way for them to receive more practical training in these lines."

He went on to request that the interested students should be told why the program was discontinued. Loma Linda offered to place and pay for a program coordinator at Andrews. The final disappointment came when their proposal was rejected out of hand. Andrews "stated very factually" that it would be impossible to give any kind of "faculty status" for any Loma Linda representative.

So, what had, for a few years, actually been a marriage between the two universities, albeit an uneasy one, ended in divorce.

More Fall-Out

The sub-specialty of church health education disappeared off the scene in 1986. Today, the subject floats vaguely through general-bulletin jargon. The SPH now has a "Christian perspective" that "forms the cornerstone of the instructional effort." This "Christian orientation and purpose" creates public health professionals whose achievements will be marked by "educational excellence."

One searches in vain, however, to recover any of the old enthusiasm of the 1970s. The time when enthusiastic conference administrators were praising the work of minister-physician teams. Nonetheless, some fifty pastors participated in the short-lived conjoint program. Most of them still remember their training as a "great asset" to their ministry, both at home and overseas. Specifically, the training brought "balance and practicality" to their work and opened doors for them that would otherwise have remained closed. These include Philip G. Semaan, a prominent author and professor at Southern Adventist University, and Matthew A. Bediako, current general secretary (2006) of the General Conference of Seventh-day Adventists

Lowell Cooper is a general vice president of the General Conference of Seventh-day Adventists and current chair of the LLU Board. He is also one of those ministers who studied public health at Loma Linda. He says: "The principles of healthful living have a very close relationship to an influence upon those of the spiritual life. I am grateful to have had the opportunity for an education that embraces both these avenues of knowledge."

Another general vice president of the General Conference is Ted N. C. Wilson (also a graduate of Loma Linda). Wilson declares: "It has been a very valuable experience to use this training in the pastoral and departmental areas of church work. Health ministry provides multiple opportunities to encourage people to live life to the fullest."

Fightings Within and Fears Without

Even worse than the failed relationship with the Theological Seminary at Andrews University were the internal dissensions within the School of Public Health itself. In the church health education program, entrance requirements tended to be low, in order to encourage ministerial students. With this perception the fat hit the fire! "Why is our public health curriculum being watered down," some academicians demanded to know. Others went so far as to say that ministers were getting preferential treatment, compared to the other public health students.

During this time, the current department chair was doing a great deal of overseas travel, along with his part-time study leave. Considerable concern arose about this "absentee leadership." Although Crawford fought valiantly to save the Loma Linda-Andrews connection, a fatal kind of vacuum had evolved. When Nelson returned to LLU in 1976, it was on a part-time basis. In 1980 he moved to Weimar Institute where he stayed until his untimely death in China in 1992. In all fairness, however, it must be said that Nelson's work helped prepare the way for the national current general interest we now find in "faith-based ministries."

Difficulties notwithstanding, a survey of SPH health evangelism activities during the years of 1971–72 gives an idea of the many ways it supported Church programs. Recognizing their full-time local teaching, the range of people, places, and programs is quite astonishing and bespeaks much energy and zeal:

1. Leo Van Dolson led a field school of health evangelism in San Jose, California (1971).
2. A team from the School of Public Health conducted a training health evangelism institute at the Mountain View Adventist Church, California (1971). About 75 baptisms resulted.
3. Many faculty assisted several successful behavior change programs at the Sunnymead Better Living Center (spring 1971).
4. Harding and Thomas led out in a "Dimension of Health" seminar at Pioneer Memorial Church, Andrews University.
5. A "Fitness and the Whole Man" team–led seminar was given in Northern California (Angwin, Napa, Elmshaven, Calistoga, St. Helena, and Yountville).
6. Wilbur Nelson conducted two field schools of evangelism, in Collonges, France, and Dublin, Ireland. Also, seminary field schools were held in Los Angeles and Plymouth, England.
7. LLU and AU offered "Take Hold of Health" to 700 church school students in Mountain View and San Jose (summer 1971).
8. The SPH faculty presented programs on health and the family at Loma Linda University Church (1971).
9. Together with the cooperation of the Ministerial Association of the General Conference (1972), the School prepared teaching materials, "Adventures in Adventist Living."
10. Mervyn Hardinge and General Conference president Robert Pierson together conducted a month-long evangelistic meeting in Idaho (1972).
11. W. J. Griffin blended health and doctrinal subjects together in a health evangelism mission at Tulane University Medical School in Louisiana.
12. At Philippine Union College new ministerial training programs were launched.

Between 1982 and 1986 the department of health education received a grant from the Sundean Foundation for $50,000 to produce the Better Living series of 10 guidebooks for conducting health education and evangelism. Dr. Joyce Hopp worked as the principal investigator on the project. Produced in both English and Spanish, the materials were distributed by the General Conference health ministries department. Dr. Kathleen Kuntaraff translated them for use in the Southern Asia Pacific Division as well as other world divisions.

As late as 1985, Donald G. King, a DrPH candidate, teamed with W. C. Scales in a "Real Truth Crusade" where 175 people were baptized. Beyond this report, the subject of health evangelism disappears off the radar screen.

The Church, of course, tends to see baptisms as a measure of the success of any enterprise. Reuben Hubbard who kept watch over the dying days of the Church health program estimated that in one field school alone, 300 people had been prepared for baptism.

Sadly, the eloquent plea of P. T. Magan saw only partial fulfillment through these painful years. "Before the end," he had declared, "every good word that God has ever spoken concerning this place" must come to pass.

This almost seventy-year-old prophecy still stands before Loma Linda University.

19

Dealing with Dependencies

Since the 1860s Seventh-day Adventists have opposed the use of tobacco, alcoholic beverages, caffeine drinks, and illegal drugs. Included, in fact, is any habit that adversely affects the mind and/or produces dependency problems.

Two major, long-standing concerns, of course, have been tobacco and alcohol.

The Smoking Gun

For most of the 20th century, smoking tobacco was recognized as the largest cause of preventable illness and deaths in the United States. More than one hundred years before modern science reached this conclusion, Ellen White denounced tobacco as "a slow, insidious but most malignant poison." It doomed young people to loss of physical strength, the dwarfing of the body, the stupefaction of the mind, and the corruption of morals (1848).

Edmond C. Jaeger, a twenty-five-year-old CME medical student, took up the burden of the tobacco problem in 1912. Not yet graduated, he lectured eloquently on the evils of tobacco in the schools of San Bernardino County and elsewhere in Southern California. The *Pasadena Star* commented on one of the colorful metaphors Jaeger employed, regarding this "well-nigh universal habit." He announced, "Cigarette smoking is all right until nature begins her foreclosure proceedings, then Beelzebub himself, prince of lawyers, can not save you. You go to the Devil's auction."

Jaeger provided an extensive list of the dismal results of tobacco use: High blood pressure, hardened arteries, apoplexy (stroke), and tendency to paralysis, as well as all of the other symptoms of old age. "Poor diet and intemperance go together ... and a man never realizes what a hold this habit gets upon him until he tries to give it up."

Jaeger quoted a professor at the University of Utah who had completed the first scientific test of the effects of tobacco and published his findings in *Popular Science Monthly*. Among his groups of students, he found that smokers had lost 10 percent of their lung capacity and had 50 percent less success in trying out for football squads. Finally, he found smoking to be invariably associated with low scholarship.

CME's publication, *The Medical Evangelist* (October 1912), speaking of Jaeger's work, earnestly expressed the hope that "many of our young men and women ... will aspire to such [smoking cessation] work and will make thorough preparation for it." This insight was far ahead of the thinking of the times, and at least 52 years ahead of the United States Surgeon General's report on "Smoking and Health" in 1964.

The Fatal Attraction

Cigarettes became readily available commercially about 1915. Before that one had to roll one's own cigarettes or smoke a pipe or cigar. The quick convenience of manufactured cigarettes brought on smoking dependency like an avalanche. In the 1930s and 1940s there began to be noticed a definite increase in the previously rare lung cancer. By the 1950s the smokers' risk of lung cancer and heart disease became obvious. The 1964 Surgeon General's report nailed the guilt firmly on cigarettes. Thousands of studies produced appalling statistics. A pack-a-day smoker had a ten-fold risk of lung cancer and a double-risk of heart disease compared with people who never smoked. Male smokers faced 22 times the risk and the women checked in at about 12 times the risk of emphysema and chronic obstructive pulmonary disease.

Loma Linda's foresight in these matters came strongly to the fore in 1937. A graduate of medical evangelism at CME, Julius Gilbert White, blazed the trail with an exhaustive search of the literature. He put together an illustrated lecture on the effects of tobacco. White promised that no question would be unanswered, that he would meet every argument, and that his program's "psychology is right." He condemned home, school, and church for failing to do their duty "to ourselves, our families, the nation, and to God" in this smoking crisis.

In the same year, an enthusiastic rally was held in the Loma Linda chapel, urging CME staff and students to combat the "almost universal intemperance" and educate children against the evils of tobacco and alcohol. The previous year, a CME alumnus had claimed that he had lectured on the health risks of tobacco to 36,531 junior and senior public high school students in the mid-Atlantic United States.

The new Physiology Building on campus (1939) pleased the faculty by providing increased space and opportunity for research work. Dr. Lester Lonergan, of the department of pharmacology and experimental therapeutics, invented a smoking machine and began to study the effects of tobacco smoke on animals. His work helped lead to what some consider to be the Adventists' greatest contribution to the fight against smoking.

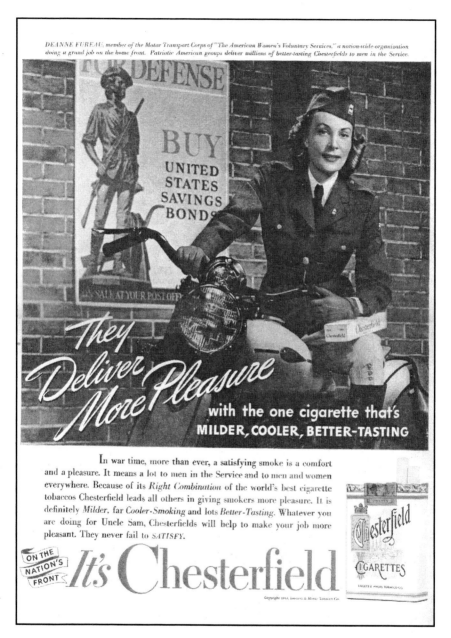

This Chesterfield ad in *LIFE* **magazine in 1942 is typical of the brazen tobacco promotion at that time.**

Two Major Achievements

Loma Linda was either directly, or indirectly, involved in both film production and the new Church developments in smoking cessation programs.

An Astonishing Film. At the General Conference Session of 1954 delegates saw the screening of the first major film to portray the relation between smoking and lung cancer, "One in 20,000." The full-color production featured Dr. Alton Ochsner, the world-renowned lung surgeon of New Orleans. By 1966 it was available in 14 languages and was estimated to have been seen by 60 million people.

Members of Parliament in Great Britain credited the film with launching the chain of events that led to the 1962 report by the Royal College of Physicians, "Smoking and Health." This publication sparked interest in the United States, and two years later the Surgeon General came out with his report. The total impact remains beyond any real estimation.

The enormous success of "One in 20,000" led the Adventist Church, with CME counsel, to produce other widely used and far-reaching "dependency" movies: "Cancer by the Carton" (1958); "Time Pulls the Trigger" (1961); and "Beyond Reasonable Doubt" (1964). The last film demonstrated Lonergan's research connecting tobacco with coronary heart disease. It also documented, for the first time, the effects of tobacco on pregnant mothers and their unborn children.

The Five-Day Plan. In the late 1950s Pastor Elman J. Folkenberg used "One in 20,000" in public meetings he conducted in London, England. At that time, he observed the large number of people who could not give up smoking, seemingly for lack of a practical plan. Upon his return to the United States, he collaborated with Dr. J. Wayne McFarland (CME '39) to develop a stop-smoking program. After testing it in New England for a couple of years, they presented it to the General Conference Session in San Francisco in 1962.

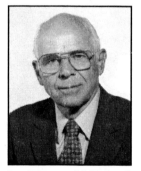

Now, training sessions for doctor-minister teams sprang up all over North America. Over three years (1962–1965) at least 20,000 smokers went through the Adventist–sponsored plan. As it rapidly spread around the world, the Five–Day Plan became the first smoking cessation program widely available. It prospered with its group-therapy approach to overcome both the psychological and physiological aspects of the lethal habit.

After the establishment of the Veterans Administration Hospital in Loma Linda, regular smoking cessation programs alternated between the VA and the local Community Hospital across Barton Road. At the 100th stop-smoking program, an SPH alumnus, Claude Turner,

J. Wayne McFarland, together with Elman Folkenberg, was the co-founder of the widely used "Five–Day Plan to Stop Smoking" which had a worldwide impact beginning in 1962.

claimed a 90 percent success rate in the 5,000 people who had taken the Five-Day Plan. That is, success measured at the end of the five days!

Attracting Research Grants

Given the long-standing interest at Loma Linda in anti-smoking research, the School of Public Health stood in exactly the right place to pull in some major research money. A two-year $215,000 grant investigated the "Psychological Factors in Self-Help Smoking Cessation Attempts" (1980). About 10,000 enrolled in that study. Judy Rausch's dissertation in 1985 confirmed the dismal fact that nurses are more prone to smoking problems than any other health professionals.

Jerry W. Lee from HLED secured a $377,968 grant from the University of California to study "The Impact of Caffeine Use on Tobacco Cessation and Withdrawal" (1990). Director of the LLU preventive medicine residency, Dr. Linda Ferry became much involved in stop-smoking research at the VA Hospital. Her work pioneered the use of buproprion as an aid to breaking the habit. She co-authored the *How to Quit Smoking and Not Gain Weight Cookbook* (2002).

Loma Linda faculty and students have participated in many stop-smoking efforts for a long time. Donald Petersen directed a large event in the anatomy amphitheater, assisted by Hardinge, Lonergan, and Charles W. Teel. Half of the 42 smokers reached their goal. Some officials in both the Church and University opposed this program—for fear that it might offend someone! (1963)

After his post-doctoral fellowship in preventive medicine at LLU, Dr. Elvin Adams worked with the United States Public Health Service Office on "Smoking and Health" (1970). An internationally recognized expert, Adams contributed much, over a period of several years, to subsequent Surgeon General's reports on smoking and health. His research on the hazards of "passive" smoking helped push through the legislation that prohibited smoking in public buildings anywhere in the United States. He also figured largely in initiating the first successful lawsuits against tobacco companies.

In 1993 LLU was awarded the Goethe Challenge Trophy as a smoke-free institution. The University became only the second institution to win this honor—and the very first in the United States.

International Influence

While the curb on smoking, particularly in the United States, appeared to be working well, the rest of the world remains substantially unenlightened. Several countries have had a fairly direct infusion of knowledge directly from Loma Linda University.

Nithat Sirichotiratana (a doctoral student in the SPH) happened to be home in Thailand in 1992. He was much pleased to find himself busy with the drafting of legislation that would stop the sale of tobacco to minors and would improve the rights of non-smokers in his country. Other SPH graduates have spent years in the stop-smoking efforts of the Bangkok Adventist Hospital. The training is largely given on the beautiful campus of the hospital's Mission Health Promotion Center at Muak Lhek, two hours north of Bangkok.

A great deal of work has also been done in China, where a man cannot consider himself a "man" unless he smokes. Barbara Choi (SPH doctoral graduate) worked in Beijing in a collaborative project of the Ministry of Health, the World Health Organization, and LLU. Funded by the Seventh-day Adventist Global Mission, this program targeted medical schools where their faculty, hopefully, would work on smoking cessation. Other participants rotated among other centers in China (Shanghai, Chungdu, Kwantung, and Xian). This is only one of many projects carried out by LLU alumni in China. A case in point is the work of Hervey Gimbel (CME '55) and his wife, who have taken anti-smoking programs to China more than twenty times and have had a tremendous national influence there.

Dr. Harley Stanton earned the Alumnus of the Year Award from the SPH in 1999 for his work with WHO advising on smoking cessation plans to the entire Western Pacific Region. In 2001–2002 Dysinger and his wife surveyed the region and reported the obvious. Loma Linda University and its graduates have more potential influence to help northern Asians get over their tobacco problems than any other group or institution.

The latest endeavor concerns a $1 million grant from NIH for Loma Linda to operate a five year program to combat tobacco-caused illness and death in Cambodia and Laos (2002–2007). The Ministries of Health in both countries are cooperating with LLU and ADRA to do research and train leaders to get control of the tobacco problem. In step with the times, the LLU Board of Trustees approved a new "certificate of tobacco control" to be offered in the School of Public Health (2002). A $150,000 grant from the Association of Schools of Public Health supports the web-site that disseminates the instruction.

Alcohol and Drug Abuse

Loma Linda hosted the first "Institute of Scientific Studies for the Prevention of Alcoholism" in the summer of 1950. Dr. Arthur L. Bietz directed this meeting, and the 95 participants heard from well-known champions of public health. The brainchild of Elder A. A. Scharffenberg, the institute continued as an annual event for twenty years mostly under the direction of Dr. Winton Beaven. These gatherings brought in a wide assortment of professions: doctors, minister, teachers, social workers, law-enforcement officers and others.

LLU medical students in the SAC Clinics (Social Action Corps—now called Social Action Community Health Systems [SACH]) assisted the dependency prevention commission of San Bernardino. In 1972 the twenty-first Institute on Alcohol and Drug Dependency at Loma Linda revealed alarming statistics. At that time it was estimated that Americans, on average, were consuming twenty tons of tranquilizers and 960 tons of absolute alcohol each day.

By the next year the SPH had attached a "Center for Dependent Behavior" to itself. Dr. Franklin Fowler, a recently discharged army officer, became the director. That year, Loma Linda received one of only two grants to study the effects of alcohol on health. Specifically, Loma Linda's grant supported a three-year study of alcohol use by 4,000 pregnant women. This project clarified what became known as the "fetal-alcohol syndrome," the bane of infants born to drinking mothers. Loma Linda researchers helped Alan Rice, a SPH graduate, obtain a $154,000 grant. When he established an alcohol treatment program at St. Helena, California, the twenty-one-bed unit was full within its first week of opening.

A Growing Field of Service

LLU's Center for Dependent Behavior (CDB) had outgrown its quarters by 1975. It moved to new facilities on Mill Street, San Bernardino. Dr. Gunter Reiss reported 60 to 80 outpatients per day. Most of them were repeat DWI (driving while intoxicated) offenders assigned by the courts. The Center employed a staff of eighteen full and part-time counselors. By 1981 the department of health science operated the CDB, which had received full accreditation two years earlier. It not only offered quality alcohol recovery programs but also served as a training facility of Loma Linda University.

Further Loma Linda research discovered a connection between diet and alcoholism. Dr. Register reported that those who drink a lot of coffee, live on nutritionally poor diets, and use strong spices could be driving themselves to alcoholic drink. A clinical drug therapist, Dr. Miller Newton, who specialized in teenage addictions and authored *Not My Kid*, lectured at Loma Linda. Jose Fuentes, of HLED, reported that his twelve years of experience showed the tests used successfully among alcoholics in western cultures were not applicable to Hispanic alcoholics.

Finally, in 1986 the General Conference of Seventh-day Adventist called a "study commission on chemical dependency and the Church" at Andrews University. Among the several LLU representatives, Hart reported the circumstances: Firstly, "the Church is recognizing a problem within." Secondly, there are definite limits to the "traditional temperance approach."

Next, LLU reorganized its well-developed dependency program in the Center for Health Promotion under the name "Clearview Alcohol and Drug Recovery Program." Dr. Mickey Ask served as the medical director and Greg Goodchild as administrator. By 1988 Ask became the

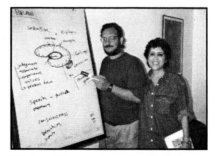

Mickey Ask, together with his wife, are shown teaching the subject of "dependencies" in Europe.

attending physician for the alcohol treatment unit at the nearby Jerry L. Pettis Memorial Veterans Medical Center, a place of great need for dependency control. He had also been named a fellow of the American Society of Addiction Medicine.

In one last "upheaval in identity," Clearview was taken over by the LLU School of Medicine. Its activities are now carried on in the department of behavioral medicine. Emphasis on dependency behavior, however, remains alive and well in the SPH and in the preventive medicine residencies where one-year fellowships are available to those who would enter a specialty that becomes more important by the day.

Dealing with dependencies has been, and continues to be, a high-priority concern of public health at Loma Linda.

20

Getting It All Together

Someone always needs to be in charge. Someone has to be at the head of the line to take both the blame and the credit. Someone has to get things done through and with people. Someone is going to sit in the corner office. Finally, the proverbial "buck" has to have somewhere to stop.

In the realm of health administration the terms "administration" and "management" are virtually synonymous. Technically, as the highest level of administration, management includes planning and design, implementation and operations, control and evaluation. All of which includes both human and material resources.

Historically, Frederick Taylor (1865–1915) is considered the father of scientific management. Working with the steel industry, he standardized parts, made work methods uniform, and invented the assembly line. Henry Ford popularized Taylor's last idea by sending his Model T down the assembly line in 1915. During this time, health education began at Loma Linda.

No doubt the discipline's best-known efficiency experts were Frank Gilbreth (1868–1924) and his wife Lillian (1878–1972). In the management of their twelve children, they carried their "time and motion studies" to a high degree of excellent organization. Not surprisingly, their humorous story, told in the book *Cheaper by the Dozen*, became a long-standing bestseller. It has passed into well over fifty languages, and several film versions have followed.

Early CME health educators took up this concept of efficiency. Always interested in the most efficient fueling and conservation of energy in the human body, J. H. N. Tindall is probably our best exemplar. From the 1920s to the 1940s he made "efficiency" the popular theme in his medical evangelism and in all of his approaches to the community.

Nonetheless, scientific management had little influence on health organizations for many years. Not until the latter part of the 20th century did Loma Linda begin to show some signs of awareness. From 1907 to 1954, physicians dominated CME's top administration—presidents and chief executive officers. When an educator first served as president, he lasted only one year before he took an overseas mission appointment. As a non-medical person he clearly felt out of place in a health institution. Although the current president, Dr. Lyn Behrens, is a physician, over the past fifty years general educators have predominated.

Do we really know what we need? The business of administration first fell to a series of accountant types, usually referred to as "business managers." Something of a "Renaissance Man," John Burden filled this position for CME's first ten years, along with being the chair of the Board of Trustees and chaplain. He also filled several other functions, as needed.

By the time the LLU School of Public Health came into being in 1967, everyone knew that trained administrators would be required. One of the core courses for the MPH was "principles of administration." Still, the question remained. What, actually, is the best training for health administrators? Opinions varied.

Should the SPH be preparing business specialists? Or did health administrators need to be equipped with general leadership skills? Should emphasis be put on training hospital administrators to serve the many Adventist institutions worldwide? Or should graduates have general health service administration skills? The debate still goes on at Loma Linda.

Public Health Practice (1967–1977)

Out of this quandary, Dr. Andrew Haynal tried to bring a few things into focus. As the first chair, he called the new administration department "public health practice." It had three sections:

1. Community (public health) administration
2. Population problems and family health, one of Haynal's own special interests
3. Preventive care administration absorbed all of the new community programs being initiated at the time

Although only the MPH degree was available, the outlook of the department constituted not only national leadership but also strong international concerns as well.

At first, the community programs carried the most clout, and leadership training went in that direction. John Scharffenberg led "Heartbeat," calling for weight control and coronary risk evaluations. Charles Thomas promoted physical fitness. Drug education, treatment and prevention programs came aboard. Many worked in the maternal, and child health programs. James Crawford arrived with a new program for public health dentistry. In short, public health practice became a catchall for any new program that did not fit in anywhere else.

Along the way, LLU undertook a relationship with the San Bernardino Social Security administration office. The students studied health and disability insurance. Lloyd Adams (the social security supervisor in San Bernardino) marveled, "This is the first time in the nation that a social security office and a leading School of Public Health have joined forces to train future health administrators."

On the Los Angeles campus, at White Memorial Hospital, Haynal provided night courses for LA County health officers. This became a forerunner of the large off-campus teaching programs yet to come (see chapter 21).

When Haynal took a two-year leave of absence to be a USAID consultant in Bangkok, Thailand, some modifications took place. The departmental name changed to health administration (HADM). The original three-part structure reshuffled into four, all of which sought to apply good business and management skills to health programs:

1. The planning, implementation, and evaluation of health care, connecting with HMO's, hospitals, health agencies, clinics, and private practice groups
2. Maternal/child health and family planning
3. International health administration
4. Dental health administration

Several commendable results accrued. The department attracted high quality students. It worked closely with the two local county public health departments, San Bernardino and Riverside. Both offices voluntarily provided teachers, advisors, and consultants for the Loma Linda program. The flip side of the coin proved to be equally beneficial. Many SPH students completed their practicums in these departments and afterwards found employment within these systems.

Family Health

The departmental emphasis in family health came about in this way. It was strong enough that for several years in the 1970s the department was called the department of health administration and family health services.

A powerful faculty of family health enthusiasts came to Loma Linda in the late 1960s. When Dr. Andrew Haynal joined the LLU School of Public Health (1967), he brought with him not only experience in general public health administration but also years of working with the Ford Foundation in family planning in India. In the same year Dr. Erwin Crawford, an OB-Gyn physician, arrived with a personal interest in maternal and child health. Dr. James Crawford was a dentist concerned with family health. Then Kay Kuzma joined the health administration department where she introduced her particular emphasis of childcare and health.

Upon obtaining a $76,700 grant from the California State department of education, Kuzma launched a unique day-care program in the Mill Street community of San Bernardino. The innovative idea was to educate parents through their children at the day care center (1974).

A few months later, LLU signed on with USAID to help the government of Tanzania develop comprehensive national MCH services. That program planted 18 regional schools in the country and trained 2,500 MCH aides. This contract turned out to be the largest of its kind ever negotiated by LLU or the Adventist Church until that time. It fed more than $2 million into the School of Public Health. At least five faculty members took part in the negotiations and management of this Africa enterprise that lasted for seven years: P. W. Dysinger (principal investigator), Richard Hart, Harvey Heidinger, and Ruth White. Joyce Hopp served as an important training consultant. (see chapter 12)

Through the years, of course, this family health program has had several different names. The content, however, has not been dissipated in any way. In 1985 maternal and child health became an area of endeavor in the new department of health promotion and education. With Christine Neish, Gail Rice, and Barbara Frye-Anderson all working hard, the program really amplified itself over the next decade. Ultimately, the LLU Board of Trustees approved a new MPH major in maternal, child, and family health. Soon, an MCH Health Services credential became available.

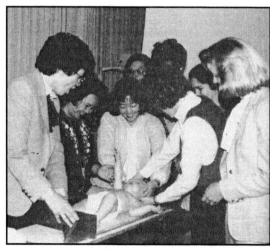

Staff and students examine an infant as a part of a mother and child health practicum.

This particular health concern has never languished at Loma Linda for one simple reason. Most people recognize the future of all society and nations depends largely on the health of mothers and their children. They are, after all, the foundation for the future.

The Era of the Master of Health Administration Degree (1978–1991)

When Dysinger became chair (1975), he saw a need to strengthen the business and management aspects of HADM. To this end, he began an earnest (and successful) "courtship" of Dr. Harold Phillips, professor of business administration at Andrews University.

The coming of Phillips (1978) brought about a new, more direct emphasis on the large network of some 200 Adventist hospitals around the world. In the 1940s and 1950s Adventist institutions had transitioned from sanitariums to acute care community hospitals. Annual retreats for HADM personnel were one of the extracurricular fine touches that Phillips introduced.

The operation of Church–owned hospitals brought in complexities. Costs for hospital care in recent years have exploded, largely it seems, due to increased specialization and ever more advanced technology. This required "third party" systems to pay for what few private patients could hope to pay. Wrestling with HMO's and sundry insurance schemes multiplied paperwork. Administrators had to shoulder much more responsibility, and, as the course of such events usually works out, they had to be paid for it.

Enter yet another problem. Since health care executives are the highest paid of all SPH graduates, naturally students have strong incentives to enter the field. How could the School find—and retain—senior faculty willing to work at LLU's wage scale? HADM has had to maintain its programs with minimal full-time faculty. It has done this by utilizing successful executives who volunteer to share their day to day experience with students in the classroom. This leads to practical down-to-earth teaching.

For hospital administrators, Phillips wanted to work on a "more focused degree," the master of health administration (MHA). It must, he said, "focus on the total well being of people" as well as business management. One of his great success stories was taking the MHA degree off campus. It began as a program for senior administrators from the 23 Adventist hospitals in the Far Eastern Division who attended classes taught quarterly in Singapore and Hong Kong. By 1987 sixteen administrators had earned their MHA degrees, and the rest benefited from significant upgrading. The president of Adventist Health Systems/Asia reported that prior to the Loma Linda MHA program, only six of the 23 hospitals had been operating profitably (1990). Three years after completion of the upgrading, 20 of the 23 were reported profitable!

In order to raise the standard, the MHA course required students to "secure and maintain membership in an approved professional society such as the American College of Healthcare Executives" (1990-1991).

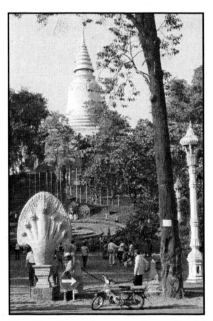

The Far East—the area where Harold Phillips took the MHA program in the 1980s, with astonishing success.

After his appointment as associate dean for administration in the School of Public Health, Phillips inaugurated a reorganization of the School (1985). For several years the SPH had no academic departments, only "programs." The result of this fancy footwork in semantics was that department chairs no longer existed. In health administration, for example, Phillips assumed program directorship for the MHA program and Walter Comm was director of the MPH program. After the turmoil of 1990, however, "departments" were reinstated.

HADM in the 1980s proudly adopted the slogan, "to administer is to minister." It aimed to be "health service oriented," not just an adjunct to a business program. Ultimately, the two degrees in HADM together covered LLU's main goals. The MHA with its one-year residency concentrated on executives and senior administrators in hospitals, managed care, and so forth. The MPH trained administrators for public health departments, nursing homes, and group medical practices.

The Current Era (1991–2004)

Several people have shaped recent trends as the chair position of HADM has frequently changed. It appears, however, that the main cause has been simply that nobody really wants to sit at the top. Everyone would prefer to work in their specialty and then talk to students about it in the classroom.

Coming from his position as public health director for the State of Delaware and with experience in medical mission work in Africa, Lester N. Wright became chair of HADM in 1991. Nationally recognized as an expert in public health policy, he brought in two new full-time instructors to help rebuild the department. On the advice of CEPH (Council on Education for Public Health), Lynna S. Belin and Dr. S. Eric Anderson joined the faculty (1992). During an interim chair position, Belin, a health economist, increased the number of course offerings and uncovered still more residency placement sites.

With a PhD in accounting, Torben Thomson became HADM chair in 1995. Under his leadership a surge in enrollment produced a new high in both morale and finance. In 1997 a new, four-year "summers only" program began. It drew students from an amazing range of foreign countries. Thomson liked to explain financial facts by means of an original metaphor. He delighted in illustrating accounting principles through use of the feedback mechanisms in the human body.

As a marketing specialist, S. Eric Anderson brought his special knowledge to Loma Linda. His success in generating more than half a million dollars in non-tuition income marked his four-year-chairmanship (1998–2002). Along with Richard Wright, Anderson implemented a new performance evaluation system. Anderson once conducted an intensive two-day training seminar for eleven Asian Adventist hospital presidents in Seoul, South Korea, calling it, "An MBA in a Day."

Other indicators show that HADM is highly motivated and now knows its identity. In 1998 Phil Carney ('95) and Joan Coggin ('87) were the first alumni to have

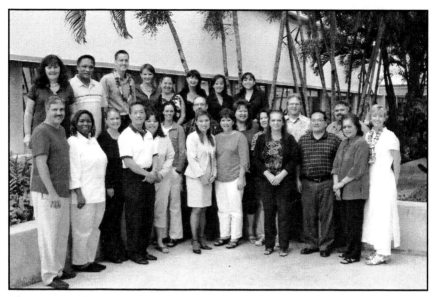

The new MBA degree program is being taught to these students in Hawaii.

$10,000 endowments established in their names. Now in an annual event, HADM, with income from its endowments, distributes about $50,000 in scholarships.

Assistant professor Bonnie Chi-Lum is editor-in-chief of the AMA's "Health Insight" website and "Kids' Health Club." LLU's students in the School of Public Health have excelled in other ways also. They ranked in the top of entries in a national contest for "generating new ideas about health care reform." In 2003 the Loma Linda team was awarded the "Making a Difference" scholarship. In 2004, HADM looked forward to establishing an innovative health oriented MBA degree program to replace the MHA.

The department of health administration remains conscious of its Adventist heritage and its commitment to the Christian perspective of wholeness. It works from a balanced base of education, research, and public health practice. The story of public health at Loma Linda often seems to be a steady juggling and manipulating of programs, finances, chairmanships, travel, course titles, and more. Instead, it may well be the simple outworking of their stated goals: To "experiment with new ideas," "bring students to their highest potential," "promote lifelong learning" for all, and to "enhance the well-being" of people around the world.

21

Discovering a New Option and Running with It

L oma Linda University hit upon a new way to educate the community in matters of health—the extended degree program. Finally, a way to earn a degree—almost without leaving home! LLU pioneered the concept and implementation of off-campus extended public health degree programs in the United States; and was the first such institution to obtain regular accreditation for such programs. Johns Hopkins University and other schools of public health quickly followed suit.

The first official off-campus teaching for Loma Linda resulted in a certificate (health education assistant), not a degree. It trained community health workers at Heri Hospital in East Africa (1956). LLU maintained this connection with East Africa until 1974.

In 1968 another project evolved nearer home. Several Los Angeles County health officers petitioned LLU School of Public Health to provide them an upgrading program. They had previously petitioned UCLA, but that university did not consider the plan to be feasible. Andrew Haynal organized a special teaching format for these health officers, and the arrangement became the University's first extended degree program.

For two years (1968–1970) LLU faculty traveled to Los Angeles, teaching intensive classes in the late afternoons and evenings. Although the first courses were held at White Memorial Hospital, the SPH also used other Los Angeles locations more convenient to the students. At that time, one term of study was required at Loma

Linda. To fulfill this obligation, the county officers arranged for one quarter to commute to the "Hill Beautiful" one day a week.

One interesting sidelight surfaced here. Being heavy smokers, some of the officer-students had a hard time refraining from lighting up while on the Loma Linda campus. Most of them, however, did manage to quit smoking before their graduation.

This first effort to take a public health degree program "to the people" was greatly appreciated by the Los Angeles County health department. Several doctors, after completing this program, were appointed district health officers or were promoted to other responsible positions in the health department. At the same time, the project stimulated good PR for the LLU School of Public Health. As an embryonic School, it needed just such a good shot in the arm.

"Come Over into Macedonia and Help Us"

In the early 1970s the School of Public Health began to receive other requests for off-campus teaching. The first came from Alberta, Western Canada, where the first two courses were offered in late 1973: "philosophy of health" and "foundations of church health education." These were well received, and this Canadian program maintained an average of twenty-five students in its classes. This pilot project ended in 1978 with eighteen graduates.

The North Pacific Union Conference of Seventh-day Adventist had been observing, and in 1975 a program was set up to serve people in Oregon, Washington, Idaho, and Montana. By 1979, 52 students received their MPH degrees at this center. Soon there were twelve centers in the United States and Canada, serving about 300 students. More sites were later added in the southern states of the United States, the mid-Atlantic area, Alaska, and Arizona-New Mexico.

Although the School of Public Health had no precedents to follow, it now had a four-year format firmly in place. (As an incentive, faculty initially received bonus money for their off-campus labors.) The program provided a wonderful opportunity for health professionals who could not easily take off a year for graduate study at Loma Linda. Suddenly, money-shortage, family, and work obligations ceased to be barriers.

Setting the Parameters

The School of Public Health set up the plan based on three foundational policies. Admission procedures would be identical, both on- and off-campus. The same teachers would teach the same courses in both places. Finally, course credit would be completely interchangeable between the two academic entities.

Sites for planting the off-campus degree programs had to be carefully negotiated. Usually, some organization or person in the field requested the service. Then a co-sponsoring organization would appoint a local facilitator who took care of the needs "on the ground" for both students and visiting faculty. Each course was packaged in a very condensed format and required pre- and post- course assignments in addition to class attendance. Teaching in the three to five day sessions some times lasted up to ten hours a day. Students were forced to immerse themselves in their study. Although otherwise the teacher-student contact was limited, the professors reported that learning in this compact time schedule worked as well, or better, than in the traditional on-campus mode. Teaching students who could immediately grasp and apply theory in their workplace turned out to be very gratifying for both teachers and students.

The regular four-year off-campus MPH program could be shortened if the student could manage to take courses at other teaching sites or enroll in some on-campus classes. In any case, some highly motivated people racked up many frequent-flyer miles as they flitted from place to place to hurry up their training.

Supervising this new way of taking health education "to the people" produced problems extending far beyond the capacity of the dean's office. After a careful examination of the new programs, P. W. Dysinger and E. A. Widmer recommended the forming of a special "service center." An office of extended programs was formed almost immediately (1976–1977). The small beginning was encouraged when the W. K. Kellogg Foundation gave LLU $188,280 to integrate the MPH degree into the family practice residencies at four hospitals in Florida, Massachusetts, Illinois, and Maryland. These programs popularized the idea of the community-based prevention work that is now common in most family medicine residencies in the United States.

These off-campus programs utilized every department in the School of Public Health. Indeed, a "generalist" (interdepartmental) program in public health best suited the off-campus format. In 2002 it took on the name of "public health practice." Although it is now available on campus, it is useful only for health professionals seeking to enrich their practice and does not serve as a foundation for a major career change.

By 2003 some 1,100 students had completed their degrees in the off-campus programs. After graduating, they moved on to a variety of leadership posts in the public health arena. North America's need for this type of training has, over time, diminished. The international interest, on the other hand, has escalated to the point where off-campus degrees are now available almost exclusively outside of North America.

More recently, off-campus learning took a very modern turn. Loma Linda announced the "executive online MPH program" in 2004. It offers a major in public health practice over a three-year period. User-friendly, the course begins with a summer-time orientation to the technology on campus at Loma Linda. At this time, one meets one's personal academic advisor, the faculty, and fellow students and gets acquainted with the library and other on-campus resources. Thereafter, for two weeks each August, students immerse themselves in intensive study on campus. For the other three terms (fall, winter, spring), the student works from his computer at home.

The targeted enrollees include physicians and dentists, nurses and dietitians, health educators and administrators, and others. The end of the course requires completion of a community practicum and report, a final, comprehensive examination, and an exit interview.

Continuing education is also associated with off-campus programs and provides short courses at workshops congruent with public health interests. These are commonly made available at conventions or other such gatherings.

International Outreach

The great success of LLU's off-campus work overseas falls naturally into four world regions—Latin America, the Western Pacific, Africa, and Europe.

1. The Latin American Programs

In the 1970s Sievert Gustavsson from Sweden served as the health director for the Inter-American Division of Seventh-day Adventist. Finding no more than half a dozen trained Adventist health workers in the entire division, he urgently appealed to Loma Linda to provide an international health training. When 113 students graduated from the first Latin American MSPH program in 1983, the division president, along with many others, marveled "how well the health message integrated with evangelism."

The program utilized three languages: the Spanish program covered Central America (Mexico, Costa Rica, Colombia, and Venezuela), while another alternated between Puerto Rico and the Dominican Republic in the Caribbean. A French group studied in Haiti. Trinidad and Jamaica shared the Caribbean English program. In every case, the subject matter was adapted to the local needs and the culture. This program was also significant as the first such program to be site-visited overseas and approved by the Council on Education for Public Health (CEPH), the SPH accrediting body.

In 1985 LLU honored Gustavsson as "University Alumnus of the Year" for his leadership in this off-campus program. A second IAD program ended in 1990 with almost 120 MPH graduates.

Currently, off-campus programs for the MPH are operating in South America, at Chile Adventist University (2001) and at the Adventist University in Peru. Both universities are on track for developing their own MPH degrees without outside assistance.

2. The Western Pacific and Asia

In 1971, P. William Dysinger stopped in the Philippines on his way home from a consultation in Tanzania. At Philippine Union College he found three men ready to enter into an affiliation with LLU, Otis Edwards, the president; Walter O. Comm; and Norman Gulley, of the Theological Seminary. They envisioned a public health teaching program on this large campus, and liaison was worked out in 1976.

Philippine Union College conducted a robust program with strong support from Loma Linda as well as from the Philippine government. The new "School of Public Health in the Philippines" gained official recognition very quickly. This came just as the college moved out of Manila to a beautiful hillside site in Silang, overlooking Lake Taal. Dr. Hedrick Edwards, and Dr. Ricardo Salamante gave strong leadership.

Then in 1986 an academic anomaly developed here, with two Adventist institutions of higher education (no more than twenty miles apart) both offering public health training. In 1978 PUC's Theological Seminary became an institution of the Far Eastern Division, and the division officers urged PUC to expand its graduate programs into other countries. People from other Asian countries had a desperate need and desire for graduate study. Negotiations with PUC, however, broke down, and a new university was formed. The original college became Adventist University of the Philippines (AUP) which serves principally the Philippines.

On a new, nearby campus the Theological Seminary combined with a School of Graduate Studies and became Adventist International Institute of Advanced Studies (AIIAS). Designed primarily to serve students outside the Philippines, it has served students from many other countries and became a General Conference operated institution in 2000.

With its MPH degree, AIIAS has delivered off-campus training to several distant places. Although AIIAS has no formal affiliation with Loma Linda, SPH faculty teach courses for AIIAS from time to time. The off-campus degree program in Cambodia was particularly significant because it offered the first public health graduate study in that country after the overthrow of Pol Pot and Communism. In 2003, Loma Linda provided a program for a new certificate of tobacco control methods. Designed for officers in ministries of health, the course was rapidly taken up by the governments of both Cambodia and Laos.

The People's Republic of China has been very receptive to LLU public health programs that coordinate with WHO and the Chinese Ministry of Health. (See Barbara Choi, chapter 19). Moreover, SPH alumni like Dr. and Mrs. Hervey Gimbel have led health education teams through more than twenty very fruitful visits to China. Stopping smoking in universities and medical schools has been a major emphasis with them.

In 1972, P. William Dysinger and his family took a sabbatical leave to help establish a health curriculum in Southeast Asia Union College in Singapore. An LLU affiliation was established in that Union which included six Adventist hospitals. Another major Asian affiliation introduced a health-training program at Pakistan Adventist Seminary and College, where a "village health worker" course was established. This training and supervision of VHW's became another LLU first.

3. African Programs and Affiliations

Loma Linda's first direct sponsored field teaching program in Africa began at Heri Hospital, Tanzania. (See chapter 11) After 25 years of successful operation, the Loma Linda affiliation with Tanzania paved the way for Loma Linda's long-standing special interest in the vast continent of Africa. Through this period of time, School of Public Health faculty also worked with other organizations such as the Trans-Africa Leprosy and Research Foundation. A leprosy survey in Zaire, Zambia, Malawi, and Tanzania was done in 1971 by Drs. Dysinger and Hart. This trip paved the way for Hart's later doctoral research in Tanzania. In the late 1980s the Adventist Central Africa University in Rwanda was in line to have a good serving of LLU public health and evangelism expertise. Then came the genocidal strife in Rwanda that destroyed that facility. It was never rebuilt.

We see that even the best of plans can miscarry, repeatedly. In 1981, a new pan-African health services office" was planned to be headquartered in Kenya. The General Conference of Seventh-day Adventist seemed to be amenable to sponsoring it. No funding came, however, and the project failed. LLU took another run at the idea in 1984. How about establishing a college of health sciences within the structure of the brand new University of Eastern Africa? Again, financial resistance scuttled the idea. As late as 1992, LLU still tried to establish an affiliation and extended degree program that would serve all of Africa. Again, that prize fruit withered on the vine.

This story, however, does have a happy ending. By 2000 the Adventist Church in Africa finally came together to find lodging for the MPH extended degree program, right where everyone knew it should have been, years earlier: at the University of Eastern Africa, Eldoret, Kenya. Finally, some quite sophisticated funding came through the Chan Shun Foundation and Swedish funds (through ADRA). This, of course, in addition to Loma Linda's own contribution.

The 65 students initially accepted into the program came from more than twenty different countries and as many different occupations. They graduated with MPH degrees in 2003. The graduates immediately transferred their new knowledge and skills directly to their institutions and communities. Africa's serious AIDS problem inspired them to become personally involved in that epidemic. Today, the future of health programs in Africa seems brighter than it has ever been.

4. European Programs

A current program in the Euro-Asia Division holds promise for Eastern Europe. In 2004 a new MPH program was funded and launched at Zaoksky Adventist University to serve the former Soviet Union and nearby countries. More than 50 enthusiastic students are enrolled in this program. Although most students are health professionals, there is a diverse group of other people enrolled.

The Crown Jewel of International Community Outreach—AHI

Adventist Health International (AHI) first became an agenda item for the LLU Board of Trustees in 1997. No action was taken. School of Public Health dean Richard Hart and Albert Whiting (from the General Conference) argued that AHI was becoming necessary because the 70 Adventist hospitals in developing countries suffered major difficulties. They had declined dramatically in their ability to serve their communities. Poor upkeep and quality of care condemned them to loss of respect in their communities. Under these conditions, young health professionals, locally or from abroad, were unwilling to commit to medical mission service in these rundown and poorly equipped institutions.

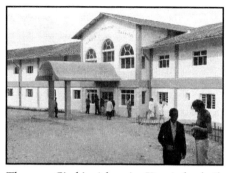

The new Gimbie Adventist Hospital rebuilt with AHI assistance.

In the next two years pilot AHI projects were undertaken, beginning with Davis Memorial Hospital, Georgetown, Guyana (1997). An example of AHI's participation is an international group from the United States, Australia, and Scotland that descended on the hospital in 2001. They upgraded the electrical system, installed dental equipment, and cheered on a class of young people graduating from a health-training program. It is reported that AHI's partnership with Davis Memorial Hospital resulted in the local church roll-call of 100 leaping to more than 1,000 members.

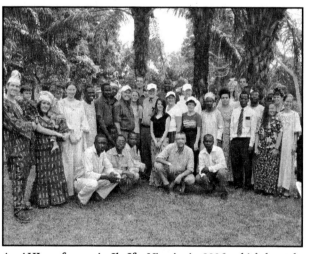

An AHI conference in Ile Ife, Nigeria, in 2006, which brought together representatives of the AHI supported hospitals in Africa to meet with Loma Linda administration, including Lyn Behrens, Richard Hart, Lynn Martell, and Don Pursley and his wife.

The second pilot AHI project

The Situations that Challenge AHI Services

1. The local Church leadership understands little about medical institutional governance and management.
2. Local church leaders can understand and accept new partnership commitments.
3. Partnership among several entities can attract external donor-support.
4. Current health-profession training and staffing is jeopardized unless hospital management and facilities are improved.
5. Although governments respect Seventh-day Adventist expertise and potential, they cannot understand the Church's "lethargy."

---

was at Gimbie Adventist Hospital in western Ethiopia. With AHI assistance, the greatly run-down Gimbie has been completely rehabilitated. There was a group of 28 SPH faculty and students who undertook a "fly-n-build" project at Gimbie in 1998. An additional eight ADRA volunteers came from the Netherlands to help. Currently AHI is actively partnering with many Adventist health care institutions in Africa, the Caribbean, India, and elsewhere.

AHI experiences caused LLU to reach several important conclusions. Their new model impacts the Adventist world Church in three ways:

1. With local churches in direct partnership with Loma Linda University, credibility is increased and more donor-support is attracted.
2. Training for health management and leadership skills is encouraged and assisted.
3. Loma Linda now offers (on request) a one-week, problem-based course on "governance." This "case-study" course benefits both church leaders and all institutional board members.

AHI holds another irrefutable doctrine: "Every health care institution must be firmly rooted in its community with concern for all aspects of development and must adopt policies that will achieve this aim." Indeed, too many hospitals in the international arena have little or no influence in their immediate communities.

Now serving more than 30 hospitals around the world, Adventist Health International has, far and away, become the largest effort yet put forth to improve the Seventh-day Adventist worldwide health care system.

22

Pushing People Out
of Their Comfort Zones

Each person has an on-going series of adventures that trails him/her throughout life. From time to time, people are urged to move beyond the secure and the predictable. In a free country, of course, those who refuse to take up the challenge are free to do so. Still, maturity and success itself depend on a willingness to escape the prison of familiarity, boredom, and mediocrity. Loma Linda's School of Public Health has long had a talent for prying people out of their comfort zones.

Back in 1905 Ellen White wrote: "The true physician ... recognizes his responsibility, not only to the sick who are under his direct care, but also to the community in which he lives." Christian health workers are obligated to serve their community. The world is, indeed, Loma Linda's community.

In 1913 twenty-four CME students organized the "Loma Linda Foreign Mission Band." The objectives aimed to "extend an interest in foreign missionary work ... [promote] a systematic study of the foreign fields ... and labor for souls." They began with study of Japan and China. Startling statistics assembled in 1923 underscored the need for missionary physicians—who at that time numbered no more 1,200 in all of the world.

Since those early days, many organized efforts have been made to keep CME students interested and involved in community service. For instance, Pastor E. Toral Seat reported from the White Memorial campus (1935) that he and the students had given about 2,500 Bible studies, "hundreds of sermons and health talks and more than 500 talks to young people." He told the Board, "We have all failed to realize in the past the great possibilities of our health program."

Physicians per Number of Population (1923)	
England:	One physician for 250
U.S.A:	One physician for 700
China:	One physician for 26,500
Bengal (India):	One physician for 42,500
Malaysia:	One physician for 300,000
Africa:	One physician for 1 million

Twin Outreach Projects: SIMS and SAC

Students for International Mission Service (SIMS) was born out of a series of interesting experiences. Dr. Clarence Stafford chaired the School of Medicine's medical mission committee and had ambitious plans for preserving CME's missionary emphasis (1955–56). He visited ten Asian Seventh-day Adventist hospitals, from Tokyo to Karachi and Manila to Bangkok. He concluded that prospective missionary doctors needed to be inspired early in their training. During their beginning service they should have access to strategically placed overseas hospitals where LLU faculty, on a rotating basis, could offer postgraduate training for both students and missionary physicians already "on location." Unfortunately, Stafford's plan never really did get off the ground, but it did prepare the way for SIMS.

In the summer of 1958, CME placed six students in mission hospitals as paramedical workers. Hopefully, the young people would gain from these mission field experiences. They did. In fact, several of them honed in on the major problems that stood in the way of recruitment and maintenance of personnel for overseas hospitals.

Although SIMS started small and developed slowly, it has always exemplified, at a very personal level, LLU's ideal of making service a lifelong process. It brings together students, faculty, and alumni to serve in some of the world's most health-care-deprived localities. Since such opportunities are rare outside of Loma Linda University, students from other universities frequently join the SIMS teams.

A fairly typical summer in 1990 produced 89 LLU students and 29 faculty members to carry out SIMS projects in 16 different countries. In 1996 sixty-five SIMS participants attended a three-day mission-training conference in northern Mexico. Thereafter, they traveled to their assignments in Nepal, Brazil, Kenya, Thailand, Korea, Hong Kong, and the Philippines.

While at first SIMS was designed to be an experiential program for medical students, people from all Schools in the University have joined in. Short mission opportunities (three to nine weeks) occur in the summers, and still more abbreviated opportunities are available during Christmas and spring vacations. LLU constantly adds new (potential) sites, and recently the number of approved locations stood above forty.

Not all projects are overseas. During the school year SIMS volunteers frequently travel to northern Mexico on the third weekend of each month. A number of projects exist in nearby San Bernardino, everything from "Adopt-a-Kid" Christmas parties to improving the scholastic skills of inner-city children through "Community Kids Connection."

Students at SIMS make many new discoveries. People in the developing world can teach much

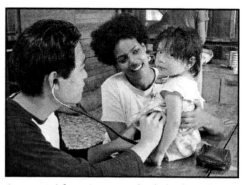

A young girl receives a medical check-up by two SIMS participants during a trip to Honduras.

about the benefits of a lifestyle of simplicity; about how to "make do and persevere;" about how to be content and savor life's rich experiences; about how to share and sacrifice; finally, to realize that all of us are more alike than different. Persons returning from a SIMS experience are never the same again. The eye-opening value of the projects cannot be over-emphasized.

SIMS leaders have always divided their time between SIMS and their "other job," whatever it is. The offices are housed in one of the historic cottages on the hill east of Nichol Hall. Philanthropic gifts provide almost all of the funding.

Social Action Corps Clinics (SAC) have been more successful and more extensive than any of the other community health programs that the School of Public Health has promoted. In 1969 a small group of medical students took note of the growing number of people in Southern California who had no financial resources. A definite humanitarian responsibility lay right here, close at hand.

With support from the University Church Seventh-day Adventist, two student-run "walk-in" clinics were opened, albeit in poorly furnished quarters and with donated equipment. As the LLU volunteer medical faculty (student supervisors) got into the work, Dr. Harvey Elder exclaimed: "I never realized how sick some of these people are!"

SAC clinics kept up their spirit and survived on the need and gratitude of the medically under-served patients. A minimum of TV and media coverage helped a little. Most of the volunteers were sophomore medical students beginning their clinical training and their supervision was by volunteer medical faculty. Initially, the Frazee Community Center in San Bernardino and the basement of the Salvation Army church in Redlands provided space for two clinics, operating between 5:00 and 11:00 p.m. three nights per week. As the volunteers graduated and moved on, the organization sometimes languished for the want of some vigorous leadership. Minimal financial support kept SAC on the borders of poverty until it was included in the United Way agencies and came to the attention of private donors.

LLU increasingly built SAC work into the medical student's curriculum. It proved to be a good place to learn the basics of physical diagnosis and cross-cultural patient care. The "working poor" who come to the clinics are predominantly Hispanic. Others have no health insurance. Many are homeless, some with chronic mental illness. At first, SAC offered free services, but the leaders found that asking for a small fee made people take themselves more seriously. Still, no one was ever denied necessary care.

An Enormous Windfall for SAC

As SAC services progressed, everyone could see that they had to find larger facilities. Not only had the number of patients increased but the volunteers who wanted to look after them also multiplied. With no capital for either purchase or rent, the volunteer leaders took turns driving around San Bernardino's ghetto area looking for abandoned buildings. The occasional gleams of hope invariably gave way to the gloom of frustration.

Then, the news broke. The government was closing Norton Air Force Base. A long shot, but the base stood only three miles away from the University campus and right next to a very large low-income area where many SAC patients resided.

Dr. Richard Hart will always recall his first visit to the base. He and Janice Crayk (part-time SAC coordinator) were shown through the clinic, a fully equipped 42,300 square foot facility. Some departments were still operating while others were packing up their equipment. Astonished, Hart and Crayk looked at the 40 examination rooms, 20 dental rooms, a clinical lab, and radiology facilities. Also a considerable amount of office equipment stood around, here and there.

"If you are thinking of applying for the building," the captain-in-charge said, "I can stop shipping equipment as soon as I have a written letter from you." Hart and Crayk stared at one another in disbelief and hastened back to the campus. They delivered the requisite letter to Norton the same afternoon.

The next day LLU entered into the pathless bog of negotiating with the government. It took many months. As expected a series of bureaucratic roadblocks impeded progress. First, the Norton clinic had to be declared military surplus. Any bona fide organization caring for the homeless would have first priority, and the University had to prove itself worthy. If enough "points" could be earned in the application, the property might be 100 percent free of charge. "By the time we were done," Hart recalls, "we had reached 110 points."

High drama ensued. A prominent figure in the transaction was George "Eddie" Hoops, who lived in Seattle and had the final signature on all property transferred to educational institutions. "You appear to be eligible," Hoops admitted, "but we need an official letter from the University Board supporting your request." Most Board members happened to be in India at that moment, attending a General Conference annual council, but in a panic of communication LLU produced the letter.

A month later Hoops announced that the government lawyers had decided that LLU, as a religious organization, could not receive government property. Then they reversed their decision a short time later. Other humanitarian groups were, of course, also on the "we-want-it" list. Months passed and LLU had no idea whether to hope or despair.

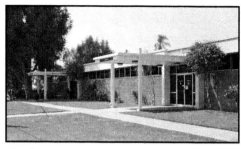

The former Air Force clinic, which is now the much used Loma Linda SAC Norton clinic.

Finally, Hoops called again. "Everything seems to be in order. I'll sign the property transfer papers next Monday."

Monday and Tuesday both came and went. No news. Then Hart received a call from an unknown person in Washington. "Eddie Hoops died of a heart attack on Sunday, while he was mowing his lawn. We thought you should know." Nothing further could be done until his replacement was installed. Moreover, the whole case would have to be reviewed again.

Long months of waiting dragged on. As the mill of bureaucracy slowly ground on, good things still happened. Interest and support among alumni and local businesses developed. Grants came in. Local city authorities expedited the necessary permits and licenses. Both SIMS and SAC became non-profit organizations within the University.

LLU, at last, received the keys to the Norton facility. In addition to the clinic building, they acquired an additional 7,000 feet of space in three trailer complexes (all set on 6.5 acres of land). Local businesses stepped forward. Home Depot, for example, donated the paint and equipment needed to refurbish the Norton buildings. The total value of the property was estimated at $6 million. On October 18, 1995, SAC Norton opened for business, beginning with an average of 60 to 70 patients a day.

Satellite SAC clinics sprang up, first in Montclair, California, under the auspices of Kaiser Permanente. Then came two in San Bernardino, "Frazee" and "Arrowhead," followed by one in Redlands. Loma Linda feels its mission is to give primary health care to the communities neighboring the University. At the same time, the clinic work provides future health professionals with values worthy of effort and commitment. Daily the students must relate to families who literally live on the edge of survival.

Perhaps the greatest reward has been the huge response from the community. The recipients of SAC services make up a sober cross-section of American inner-city life: trigger-happy gang members; babies born with a five times greater chance of being murdered than going to college; young mothers moving from room to room

---

The Menu for Loma Linda's SAC Clinic Services

- All types of physical exams   - X-ray and laboratory services
- Pre-natal services   - Immunizations
- Pharmacy   - Dental care
- Nutrition counseling   - Health education
- Behavioral (mental) health problems
- Neurological and rehabilitation services
- Individual, family, and group counseling
- Alcohol and drug treatment services
- Therapy: physical, occupational, and speech
- Diagnosis and treatment for both acute and chronic illness

---

with their growing brood, trying to avoid eviction; thugs dealing in drugs and trading bullets in order to get rich; and the hard-working down on their luck. All gravitate to the SAC clinics trying to regain their hope and their dignity.

In this environment, LLU students daily confront the challenges of relating with families who literally live on the edge of survival, and yet are equally precious in the sight of God as are Loma Linda faculty and students. "We want our students," Hart explains, "to feel comfortable and able to respond to these challenges in fairness and love …. All this behavioral pathology is not the choice of those caught up in it, but is the result of sin and the dysfunctional relationships sin has produced."

In 2003, Dr. Richard Hart was chosen, on behalf of SAC, to receive the "Inland Empire Leader of Distinction Humanitarian Award." People everywhere had no trouble understanding why he and SAC so richly deserved the honor. Who could count the number of people he had helped push out of their comfort zones in order to take "health to the people" around the world.

23

The Resurrection of a Good Idea

The old "Sanitarium idea" had always called for long-term care, measured in weeks or months, not days or hours. Its purpose? To reinforce good health habits and promote healthful lifestyle change.

Early in the 20th century medical education took a powerful new turn. The new emphasis on the basic sciences (anatomy, physiology, biochemistry, and microbiology), inspired largely by the Flexner Report, tended to encourage specialization and sub-specialization. Like everyone else, graduates from the young College of Medical Evangelists followed the trend and gravitated to Vienna and other centers of specialization for post-graduate study. The first American Specialty Board established itself in 1916: ophthalmology was the first recognized specialty. Today, the American Boards recognize more than sixty specialties and sub-specialties.

The usefulness of specialties notwithstanding, the fall-out has resulted in severe "depersonalization" in patient care. At the extreme, the patient is reduced to being simply a number in a file. Instead of treating people who are sick, physicians tend to see "problems" of heart, respiratory, or kidney disease. Like technologists and engineers, doctors tend to care for cancer "cases." They remove or replace defective body parts or try to find powerful, new antibiotics. Then, a whole spectrum of other lethal problems evolves. Rene Dubos confesses that "modern medicine frequently creates new diseases as rapidly as it subdues old ones."

Along with all of her academic counterparts, Loma Linda has largely been built on the belief that disease is mainly the result of outside, hostile forces that must be eliminated. Patients need to have something done to them by their physicians. Happily, a new paradigm is now gaining favor. People need to take more self-responsibility and recognize that disease derives from the poor choices people make in lifestyle habits, something they do to themselves. As much as 70 percent of illnesses fall into this category, according to the United States Surgeon General, and risk assessment and lifestyle education must be the potent, new tools. The two philosophies severely clash.

Yet, there is really "nothing new under the sun." In 460 BC Hippocrates said: "Before undertaking the treatment of a patient, learn his habits and make your treatment according to his habits."

The "Sanitarium idea" now steps into the foreground once more.

Another Lengthened Shadow

Early students and faculty at CME will remember Pastor J. Lee Neil (1908–2000) as the white-haired gentleman attending School of Public Health functions. Usually he could be found in the kitchen with Allan Magie preparing food for conventions, graduation celebrations, and so forth. It might be easy to miss the fact that Neil was a kingpin in lifestyle education.

Pastor Neil's basic Adventist training came from Walla Walla College and St. Helena Sanitarium. His qualification as a medical evangelist came out of the large, highly successful field training school of J. H. N. Tindall and W. D. Frazee (see chapter 4). Ordained to the ministry of the Adventist Church in 1934, Neil served in several conferences, Arkansas-Louisiana, New Jersey, and Potomac. Everywhere they went, Pastor Neil and his wife worked tirelessly in various types of medical missionary work, bringing ministers and doctors together wherever possible.

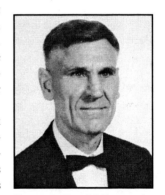

Early in his work in Louisiana, Pastor Neil met Rex and Maudine Callicott, who had a successful cookie-baking business in Baton Rouge. An astute businessman, Rex had also added land investments and oil to his bakery business. Under Neil's influence, the Callicotts rejoined and strongly supported the Adventist Church. In times to follow, they donated more that $5 million to various Church projects, mostly at Neil's behest, including the seed money to help start the Seventh-day Adventist Ministerial Association's "Preach" project.

Pastor J. Lee Neil was the prime facilitator of the movement, beginning in the 1960s, towards new Adventist lifestyle programs.

A Plethora of Projects

In 1950 Pastor Neil, while in the Potomac Conference, set up a non-profit organization, Medical Ministry, Inc. (The name changed in 1980 to Adventist

Ministries, Inc.) By the 1960s Neil had been freed from local pastoring in his conference to promote health evangelism full time.

In 1962 he landed a "big fish." He persuaded the governor of Louisiana to sell the state-owned resort of Hot Wells to the Adventists for "a new type of health institution." He summoned Drs. Mozar and Farag from Loma Linda to examine the situation. "The division of public health and tropical medicine," Mozar replied, "would be glad to adopt Louisiana as a place for a pilot project in research." It would assist those "desiring help in physical fitness and habit correction."

Enthusiasm abounded. Rex Callicott and his affluent partner, John Barton, sat in the governor's office and assured him: "Finance will not be an obstacle." A bid for the purchase was placed. Farag exclaimed, "The Lord will honor your unselfish effort and that of Elder Neil. Whatever happens to the Hot Wells proposition, [your] thorough work ... will not be in vain."

Along the way Neil had connected with influential local people in Louisiana. For instance, Dr. Alton Ochsner, founder of the Ochsner Clinic in New Orleans. (He starred in the Adventist film, *One in 20,000*). He supported the Hot Wells project as a "splendid thing" and "a real asset to our State." In the end, however, the governor's plan to sell Hot Wells was withdrawn—due to political pressures.

In 1964 J. Lee Neil attended the First International Conference on Preventive Cardiology, which convened at the University of Vermont in Burlington. For five days he listened to world-famous specialists proclaim that the answer to "our greatest killing problem (cardiovascular disease) is not pills but prevention, not clinical but educational." The pastor came away more fired up than ever over the "new concept" of lifestyle medicine.

Scripture commands "undo the heavy burdens and let the oppressed go free." Neil felt absolutely possessed "to break every yoke." Just at this stage, a kindred spirit, Dr. P. W. Dysinger, returned to Loma Linda from his two-year mission at Heri Hospital in Africa.

Dysinger was more than happy to help plan and assist a ten-day physical fitness institute that Neil organized at Fountainebleu State Park, near New Orleans (1965). About twenty people attended this, the first Adventist conditioning

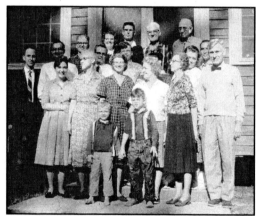

The first new Adventist lifestyle change program—a physical fitness institute at Fountainbleu State Park in Louisiana in 1965. Dysinger is on the left, Neil on the right.

project. At the end testimonials were enthusiastic; from non-Adventists working with their tobacco addiction; from others who struggled with obesity and diet; from the helpers and staff who learned new methods.

Dysinger immediately recognized the great potential of this pilot program, but he pointed out two important considerations. What about the difficulty people had in leaving their work, even for just ten days? Also, he wanted to "aim directly at [addressing] specific problems"—not general prevention. He eagerly anticipated the part that LLU could have in developing better methods and materials for health education.

Actually, the influence of this first, small Adventist lifestyle program spread around the world, sometimes with an "electrical effect!" Dr. S. A. Kotz wrote from Australia that the institute coordinated well with what he had been thinking but had been unable to "bring into focus."

Maintaining Connections

With his typical entrepreneurial skill, J. Lee Neil maintained close contact with at least four influential men he had met at the Vermont preventive cardiology conference.

Dr. George C. Griffith, professor of medicine at the University of Southern California, counseled Neil: "I do hope that the LLU will strongly support such a [conditioning] center." As president of the American College of Cardiology, his opinions carried weight. Dr. T. K. Cureton, professor of physical education and director of the physical fitness research laboratory at the University of Illinois, announced: "I have long known of the fine work done by Adventist's in the direction of more healthful living, and I would give my cooperation to a well-defined project carried out by this group."

Dr. Paul Dudley White (cardiologist to several United States presidents and emeritus professor of medicine at Harvard University) recalled a 1966 meeting with Neil and other Adventists: "[I am interested] in their hope to establish health centers in this country and abroad." Then he added a word of caution: "It is very important to make a study of such health centers to see how much improvement, longevity, and good health may come from them."

Some consider emeritus professor of experimental medicine at the University of Vermont, Dr. Wilhelm Raab, to be the father of "preventive cardiology." An interest that led directly to the "conditioning concept" in the United States. When Raab established his "Preventive Heart Reconditioning Foundation, Inc.," Paul Dudley White became the honorary president and Maria von Trapp (of *Sound of Music* fame) the vice president. Other distinguished preventionists joined in. These included Drs. Irvin H. Page, Jeremiah Stamler, Hans Kraus, and Hans Selye (of stress control fame). With his usual vigor, Neil maintained close contact with the Preventive Heart Reconditioning Foundation.

Indeed, Raab confided to Pastor Neil, "Meeting with you again ... was an extraordinary pleasure for me ... and gave me a great moral lift after years of frustration." He hoped that "at long last something really worthwhile will be done in the field of health preservation." Neil sent him copies of *"Life at Its Best"* and *"A Century of Miracles,"* and Raab praised such a "vivid … and convincing impression of the philosophy and achievements of your church."

In fact, as a result of Neil's report of the first preventive cardiology conference, Dr. Alan Harmer, medical director, Herbert Atherton, business manager, and Petra Sukau of Wildwood had already visited and studied "conditioning centers" in Europe. They carried with them letters of introduction from Drs. Raab and Paul Dudley White. This visit inspired them to begin a similar program in Wildwood, Georgia—the first such inpatient lifestyle program operated by Seventh-day Adventists.

As far back as 1939, Raab had given a series of lectures at Loma Linda, and he desired to keep that connection intact. A later comment from Raab would prove to be painfully ironic. "No matter how difficult and long the way toward realization of your planned center may be," he said, "it makes me feel good that energy and enthusiasm are at work in your group to get things really under way." Just how that energy fared is the story of our next chapter.

Invitation to Innovation

In 1966 Raab and White held a second International Conference on Preventive Cardiology, this time in Stowe, Vermont. This time Neil brought five other Adventists with him. After one of Paul Dudley White's legendary three-mile morning walks, the Adventists had a "cozy conference" with both Raab and White. Intent on spending his life in preventive cardiology, Dr. Richard T. Walden, associate dean of the new School of Public Health at LLU, asked for advice. Raab and White suggested the best conditioning centers in Europe that he should visit and discussed other matters relating to the starting of conditioning centers. "Their programs," the doctors said, "are in many respects like what Adventist sanitariums used to be."

Having made his survey during the winter of 1967–1968, Walden escorted three significant people to see what he considered the eight best conditioning centers in Germany, Austria, and Switzerland. Those people were Dr. Mervyn Hardinge, dean of the School of Public Health, and his wife, Margaret, and Mr. Rex Callicott.

Leadership in the development of conditioning (lifestyle) centers had fallen squarely in the lap of Loma Linda University. "All systems go" appeared to be the watchword.

24

Makeovers in the Extreme

The current passion for "extreme makeovers," of course, grows out of the innate human belief that our lives can be improved upon. Millions of people give themselves over to cosmetic surgery and dentistry, liposuction and tummy-tucks, and new wardrobes—to say nothing of customized make-up and hair styling. These surface enhancements are quite ephemeral compared to the Loma Linda idea of a makeover. One that involves education and decisive changes in lifestyle.

Studying the Models

Conditioning centers first appeared in West Germany in the late 1940s and early 1950s and were designed to counteract depredations of affluence and inertia on the human body. "Conditioning," or reconditioning, is the improvement of physical fitness, cardio-respiratory function and the strengthening of the immune system. It results from the practice of organized exercise, diet, recreation, health education, and social support.

Because diseases of the cardiovascular system were proliferating all over the Western world, a group of American physicians accepted an invitation from the federal government of West Germany to visit their reconditioning centers in 1963. A social insurance law in West Germany in 1957 provided for any worker to stay at a conditioning center for up to six weeks, upon the recommendation of a physician. Twenty such centers already existed at that time.

What the Americans found has a familiar ring to it today. Sixty years ago, however, these facilities were very avant-garde. Situated in isolated, rural areas, they provided simplicity of environment. The staff, including physicians and a social worker, offered a whole smorgasbord of benefits: health education and group sessions, phys-iotherapy/hydrotherapy, physical exercise, wholesome diet, daily recreation, and rest. More than 75 percent of the clientele improved their cardio-vascular systems, and many became symptom-free during their treatment. Improvements lasted for a year or more in at least half the guests.

Without waiting for scientific proof of their methods, the Germans had simply plunged into their reconditioning programs. Tradition, clinical experience, and com-mon sense supported them, they said. Happily, industry (and the labor unions) found that absenteeism was much diminished and that their production and the economy improved. Also, the reconditioned employees were "more apt to postpone premature" retirements.

Dragging Anchor

From its beginning, Loma Linda's School of Public Health emphasized lifestyle medicine. In 1966, the public health faculty proposed an exciting research project that could have involved the entire University. They proposed a multi-disciplinary research program in preventive cardiology to fight degenerative heart disease, the largest single cause of death in the United States. The German conditioning centers, the Framingham Heart Study, and Loma Linda's own Adventist health studies all supported the SPH's ambitious proposition. The practical application of the plan would be the creation of an institution where disease-prone people could spend three to six weeks in a reconditioning program. The School of Medicine could carry out clinical evaluations. The School of Nursing could help staff the institute. All of the resources of the Schools of Allied Health Professions and Public Health could be uti-lized in implementation and basic and applied research.

The accumulated scientific evidence for such an enterprise would surely mobi-lize everyone for action!

Not so. Inertia set in, and for reasons never really clarified.

The next year, Dr. Mervyn Hardinge, the first dean of SPH, reflected on the sit-uation. "The teaching of healthful living," he declared, "must be made practical." That is, Loma Linda needed to develop its own conditioning center. "Other schools of public health cannot offer any real, basic philosophy of health," he went on. "Therefore, our health education program can and should be better than any other in the world."

The wheels of progress rotated just an inch or two. The lack of University sup-port caused the initial idea to perish on the launching pad.

Six years later Hardinge still had a teaching conditioning center high on his list of priorities. He urged his case to members of the University Board and the General Conference administration. "If we could have a conditioning center, we could be a model for our physicians and health-trained workers worldwide." Indeed, he envi-sioned such an institution as a "catalyst for our entire [church] work." Loma Linda

School of Public Health was, in fact, the only Church-supported school of public health in the world. It became painfully evident, however, that some in the University remained less than enthusiastic about the project.

Even after Dr. Hardinge survived a near-fatal heart attack (1976), he never slowed down in his efforts to create a conditioning center. This time, he took a different line. Since the healing ministry must be a tool for the gospel ministry, perhaps the School of Public Health should transfer to the campus of Andrews University in Michigan. Lively discussion ensued, but finally most Board members favored leaving the school where it was.

That idea also sank into oblivion.

One Error Too Many

Somewhere, deep at the core, bureaucracies have a morbid tendency to self-destruct. They tie themselves up with miles of red tape and then shoot themselves in both feet. All of this to the utter frustration of their constituencies, the public in general, and many of the participants themselves. Dr. Hardinge now found himself at the center of just such a chaotic situation. The tale would unfold in a series of unbelievable episodes.

Hardinge's busy mind, of course, went on planning. A young, up-and-coming internal medicine resident with an interest in cardiology, Dr. Richard Hart, held an assistant professorship in the School of Public Health. An ad hoc committee saw him as a progressive leader who could bridge the gap between clinical and preventive medicine. They talked about a "marriage" between medical and SPH students—hopefully to be followed by a long, happy honeymoon. In early 1979 the prospects looked hopeful.

Enter now a new player on stage, the wealthy businessman and philanthropist Rex Callicott (member of the LLU Board of Councilors). Mervyn Hardinge had long ago told him all about the dream of a model conditioning center at Loma Linda. In fact, in early 1968, they had visited eight European conditioning centers, each one enhanced by its lovely rural setting. Some time later, Mervyn called Callicott. "Are you ready to talk to the president of LLU?"

"Most certainly," he replied unequivocally. Callicott boarded a plane for California.

In due course, Hardinge appeared at the president's door. "Mr. Callicott is ready to make a financial offer. Are you interested?"

"Of course!" (Who wouldn't be, one might ask).

"Mr. president," Callicott leaned forward to emphasize his point. "For many years I have been interested in giving a conditioning center to your School of Public Health. I will build it. I will equip it. And I will endow it."

A golden moment! Yet, the impossible happened. Callicott never received a word of thanks, then or later. The offer to the University died.

By the time the next president had taken office, Hardinge had found a wonderful

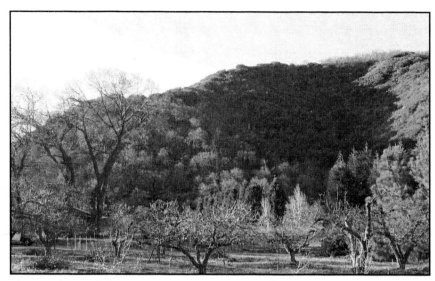

The Snowline apple orchard in the foreground with Pisgah Peak in the background. It was considered in the 1970s as an ideal site for Loma Linda's training/research center for lifestyle change programs.

property, Snowline Ranch, at 5,000 feet elevation in Oak Glen, just 30 minutes' drive from Loma Linda. The situation seemed ideal. By now the SPH had even managed to save $300,000 towards a Center. The University already owned Pisgah Peak behind the apple orchard now up for sale. The mountain had no water and no access, except through the orchard. Now, for a bargain of $175,000 the orchard could be bought and the whole property opened up. The president and another University official visited the property.

A few days later, the president called Hardinge. "Well, have you bought the property?"

Ever respectful, Hardinge replied, "I can't buy property. The Board has to approve it."

"No, no!" the president soothed. "You have the money, and you don't need Board approval. I shall instruct the Foundation to purchase it."

A man assigned to accomplish the transaction promptly followed up the conversation. "Just tell me what you need."

"Well, be sure to get the water rights and shares." Emerging from the bliss of a dream coming true, Hardinge thought fast. "Oh, yes, and get as much of the orchard equipment as possible," he added.

A few days later, the man called again. Hardinge was about to leave for Australia. "It's all done," the caller chortled. "We've signed the contract." Hardinge breathed a prayer of thanks and departed for Australia.

Upon his return home, two weeks later, he received a call from the very irate owner of Snowline Ranch. "What do you mean, backing out of the deal like that?" The voice fairly bristled with hostility.

Frozen in shock, Hardinge felt his heart drop all the way down to his feet. "Excuse me! I've been away for two weeks, and maybe I have jet-lag, but I don't know what you're talking about."

"You mean that you don't know that your president wrote a letter saying the deal's off?"

"You're kidding!"

"I am not kidding." The furious caller went on. "You know, I could sue your institution for this."

"I think you could," Hardinge replied humbly.

Records show that the Board decided the price was too high. They seemed to have overlooked two important facts: a donor stood ready to foot the bill, and without this purchase Pisgah Peak would remain virtually worthless property.

Some time later, the president became inexplicably interested in the conditioning center again. "Do you think, Dr. Hardinge, that Brother Callicott is still interested?"

Feeling his face burn again, Hardinge replied carefully. "I don't know, but I can ask him."

Forthwith, Rex Callicott returned to the same office, same desk, but a different president. He reiterated his first offer. "I have already given away large sums of money that I had planned for this project, but I am still interested. I'll carry through."

History then repeated itself, down to the last detail. Once again, not a word of thanks nor a letter of acknowledgement.

Meanwhile, LLU got a new public relations man from Andrews University. He approached Hardinge. "I understand that you know Rex Callicott. He helped us a great deal at Andrews. Didn't he come here and make some offers?" Hardinge related the sad story. "Why, I've never heard of such a thing in my life," the PR man exclaimed.

"That's what happened," Hardinge said doggedly. "I have virtually been on my hands and knees begging the president to acknowledge Rex's offer and thank him for it. I can't get a word out of him."

With a glint in his eye, the PR man declared: "Callicott will get a letter, I promise you."

"And how will you do that?"

"Easy. I'll write maybe twenty letters and lay them all before him at once for his signature. Callicott's will be one of them." Thus, the patient philanthropist actually did get a thank-you letter.

Then opportunity knocked again! The largest apple orchard in Oak Glen, Los Rios (312 acres), came up for sale. The persistent Hardinge approached two donors this time, the long-suffering Rex Callicott and Dr. Reuben Matiko from Canada. After walking over the property, the men devised a painless way to buy it. Within days, Hardinge gave the owners a down-payment of $500,000 for Los Rios. Next week the papers would be signed.

Before that could happen, however, Hardinge got a call from one of the owners. The man was half crazed, and the phone lines almost ignited with the heat. Hardinge had no idea what it was all about, but he had a sickening feeling that he could guess.

"You mean you don't know?" the man raged. "Your president has cancelled the deal."

Engulfed in disappointment, Hardinge could only say, "This is a unilateral action. I thought everything was finished." The roof had caved in again on the idea of a conditioning center for the School of Public Health.

Next, the president conceived of a compromise of his own. Why not have the conditioning center right on campus? Building a 30-room motel accommodation on the hillside below the School of Public Health (Nichol Hall) could also be a great money-saving move. The pool and other facilities were already in place in Nichol Hall. A committee vaguely recommended proceeding with the project, "as funds are available." This time, however, no donors came forward to sponsor a conditioning center in the middle of Loma Linda's heavily urbanized campus.

Mervyn Hardinge and J. Lee Neil made one final effort to establish a lifestyle center. The proposed "Living Oaks" [Southern Sanitarium], stood on 200 acres in southern Louisiana, between Baton Rouge and New Orleans. Complications to this proposal ensued. Hardinge now felt it was time for him to retire from the field. By now the negotiations for a conditioning center had been going on for seventeen years. Hardinge, no doubt, felt that he had been scrambling for "scraps under the master's table" for long enough. Time had run out.

25

Taking Up the Slack

Although Loma Linda never secured its own lifestyle center, others stepped into the breach. These independent institutions could justifiably be regarded as revivals of the old Adventist tradition of the sanitarium. They were owned and operated by Seventh-day Adventists, and most of them were staffed by Loma Linda graduates.

At least twelve centers come to mind.

St. Helena in the Napa Valley of California is the oldest Seventh-day Adventist-owned health institution in the world. Although it is now a regular community hospital, it began as a rural retreat, a "sanitarium." It has long specialized in alcohol and tobacco addictions, as well as individualized programs for health improvement. For a number of years, Dr. John A. McDougall was probably their best known staff physician.

Wildwood Sanitarium and Hospital in Georgia began in 1941 with three men of vision, Neil Martin, W. D. Frazee, and George McClure. It subsequently evolved into the first new Adventist lifestyle center in 1971. J. Lee Neil had encouraged the Wildwood administration to visit the best conditioning centers in Europe and this inspired new ventures. Lifestyle-change programs have been going on at Wildwood ever since. The training of a new type of natural medicine practitioner is presently being pioneered at Wildwood.

Weimar is in the foothills of the Sierra Nevada Mountains, California. A leap of faith began with the purchase of a former state-operated tuberculosis sanatorium. The staff based their program on the eight natural remedies advocated by Ellen White: nutrition, exercise, water, sunshine, temperance, air, rest, and trust in God. The copyrighted acronym for their treatment package is NEWSTART. Weimar's pioneering influence on conditioning centers has been felt all around the world. Again, many of the staff are LLU graduates.

Uchee Pines, Alabama, is a non-profit health education and small conditioning center (14 guests). In 1971, the founders, Drs. Calvin (LLU MPH '69) and Agatha Thrash focused on nutrition, graded exercise, hydrotherapy, and other natural treatments. Uchee Pines is also active in training medical missionaries in the use of non-drug therapies.

Black Hills, South Dakota, was founded by SPH graduates. Its magnificent natural setting has long been considered sacred ground by the Native Americans there. A day's agenda can be created out of many options: water therapy, cooking class, consultation with a doctor and/or an exercise physiologist, and swimming. This, plus vegetarian meals, massage, and instruction in stress management.

Lifestyle Center of America, Oklahoma, is one of the newest Adventist lifestyle centers. Beautifully equipped and furnished, it seeks to be on the cutting edge of organizations designed to prevent and reverse common Western degenerative diseases (such as diabetes). Again, most of the medical staff has had training at Loma Linda University School of Public Health. LCA has been approved for residency training of Loma Linda's preventive medicine residents.

Eden Valley Institute is located at the foot of the Rocky Mountains near Loveland, Colorado. It has operated an active lifestyle center for a number of years, following the NEWSTART approach. It is also known for its organic gardening and training in agriculture and for its foreign mission training program.

CHIP (Coronary Health Improvement Project) was established by Dr. Hans Diehl, in 1988. It has been the largest and most successful community oriented outpatient lifestyle approach, so far. His pioneering efforts with Nathan Pritikin and Dennis Burkitt led Diehl to develop this program. It usually operates as a 4-week (16 session) lifestyle change program. The program currently operates under the Lifestyle Medicine Institute at Loma Linda or under the Adventist CHIP Association headquartered in Sulphur, Oklahoma.

The LLU conditioning concept has now migrated overseas. *Eden Sanitarium* is located about two hours northeast of Seoul, South Korea. With 200 beds, it is currently the largest Adventist Church operated lifestyle center in the world. Specializing in cancer treatment, the center also operates group programs to prevent and treat

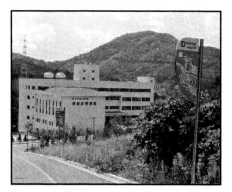

Two hours from Seoul, Korea, is the largest Adventist owned lifestyle center in the world, Eden Sanitarium.

common degenerative diseases through diet, exercise, hydrotherapy, and other simple modalities.

Two other important Asian lifestyle centers are operated by Adventist hospitals in Taiwan and Thailand. For a number of years, Mission Hospital Bangkok has operated a lifestyle center where a NEWSTART-type program is available. In addition to being a popular option offered to Thai people, it has also provided special programs for Koreans and for Chinese from Hong Kong. It has a lovely facility at *Muak Lhek,* in a beautiful rural area two hours north of Bangkok.

Taiwan Adventist Hospital operates the *Yu-Chi Health Education Center* in central Taiwan in the resort area near Sun-Moon Lake. It is a beautiful well-equipped 45-room guest facility that also follows the NEWSTART plan. Since the previous facilities were destroyed in a 1999 earthquake, the present facility has functioned since 2001.

Herghelia Institute of Health has been operating in Romania since 1986. As an English-language lifestyle treatment center, it provides 11- and 18-day programs throughout the year, with 35 to 40 guests in each session. It also operates a 12-month lifestyle counselor training school. The institute was established and administered by Dr. Nicholae Dan and his wife, Valentina, both of whom are LLU School of Public Health graduates.

Lacking its own center, LLU has depended on these related institutions for field experience. Research has shown the lifestyle interventions used in these Adventist operated institutions may be even more effective than the popular DASH (Dietary Approach to Stop Hypertension) program created by the NIH National Heart, Lung, and Blood Institute.

The current Adventist lifestyle intervention research asks questions like "How do health beliefs and spiritual input affect outcomes? How can we better control medication management? How can randomized trials (with good controls) be organized within these programs?"

Although difficult to evaluate, many of these questions might have been answered long ago, if the School of Public Health had been able to proceed with an inpatient-conditioning center. Today, LLU would give a king's ransom for one of those Oak Glen properties complete with a conditioning center. All paid for and endowed.

In recalling this long, sad episode, Hardinge says: "I see so many opportunities that the Lord has given, and how we have failed Him so many times." Perhaps a good Jewish proverb is instructive here. "God holds us responsible not just for our sins but also for the pleasures and gifts He gave us that we refused to accept."

Although Loma Linda's work in preventive medicine did not evolve in the way that Dr. Mervyn Hardinge envisioned, the pressure never really let up. Eventually the School of Public Health and the School of Medicine did combine to produce other new preventive programs, complete with the always-essential academic degrees.

26

Lifestyle Medicine Can Work

W hat the early College of Medical Evangelists really wanted to do was produce lifestyle-change specialists. Unfortunately, it was 60 years ahead of
the times. Medical philosophy and practice in the 1910s and 1920s saw
little potential for lifestyle change. As we have seen, traditional medicine won out at
CME, and efforts in dietetics also faced great difficulties.

Nonetheless, starting with John Harvey Kellogg at the Battle Creek Sanitarium,
there have always been a few voices crying in the wilderness. The roll-call is actually
a long one and includes names like the Drs. Daniel and Lauretta Kress, J. Wayne
McFarland, Lester Lonergan, and Marion Barnard, to cite but a few.

Defining Lifestyle

The launching of Loma Linda's School of Public Health in 1967 forecast its function as the flagship of all "conditioning endeavors." Charles Thomas' physical fitness
program and John Scharffenberg's "Heartbeat" programs were both born in what was
first called the public health practice department. Biostatistics and epidemiology documented the success of lifestyle change in the Adventist Health Studies.

These good works, however, could not achieve the status that lifestyle medicine
needed. A new doctoral program had to be developed. After intense study and preparation on the part of the faculty, the doctor of health science (DHSc) degree program
came into being in 1972. Although its basic science foundations resembled that in
conventional medicine, it went a step further. This new health promotion specialist
would be expert in teaching, research, in identifying risks, and then counseling the
patient about lifestyle changes. He/she would also design and market programs, all
the way from the church to industry.

From the start, some of the medical faculty watched the new doctoral program with a keen suspicion. Clearly, these new specialists would surpass regular doctors in their knowledge about nutrition, exercise, addictions, stress control, and other preventive programs. A little jealousy here, maybe? What if these new doctors felt qualified to do what "regular" physicians do? Would their heads get too big for their hats? A program so far ahead of its time would, naturally, arouse fear and opposition.

Academic Training

When the doctoral degree program was officially inaugurated in 1972, there were twenty students ready to enroll. Consistently, Dr. Hardinge admonished these new doctors not to consider themselves as regular medical practitioners. Instead, they were to be the kind originally envisioned in the beginnings at Loma Linda as "evangelistic-medical practitioners" or "medical evangelists."

Seven years later, outside observers and the accrediting organization pronounced the DHSc degree to be a strong program and on the cutting edge as one of the most "innovative" programs in existence "to address the specific needs of health." An evaluation of the first 68 graduates in 1979 revealed that the largest number (46 percent) were working for Adventist institutions or programs. Twenty percent had government or university employment; and most of the rest were in some type of private practice.

A new department of preventive care was developed as the home for the DHSc "clinically oriented health educators." Although chairmen and program-descriptions changed with amazing speed, Hardinge's presence provided continuity. New names, however, cropped up: Alan R. Magie, Albert Whiting, Raymond West, Richard Hart, and others.

During his years of leadership, Richard H. Hart reoriented the School of Public Health's innovative doctoral degree. The title, "DrPH in Preventive Care," indicated an intentional effort to make the lifestyle change program more acceptable (1991). Interest in this lifestyle-change doctoral program remains satisfyingly strong to this day.

Two Mixed Marriages

Loma Linda University was the first school to arrange two unique academic marriages. LLU combined the regular MD with the MPH degree. Likewise, the DDS (doctor of dental science) could also join with the MPH. Richard Hart had unofficially broken ground back in 1968 in his personal academic program. This enabled him to be the first in the United States to complete concurrently both the MPH and MD degrees (1970). The next year a number of medical and dental students pressed for an official "combo" degree. Curiously, largely through the influence of James Crawford, more dentists than physicians took up this early opportunity. Although these combined degrees are now common in many North American universities, Loma Linda led the way.

By applying all of their electives to the study of public health, this relatively simple plan enabled the students to earn the minimum required for the MPH. The School of Medicine and SPH meticulously spelled out the requirements, and candidates were required to place in "the upper half of their medical class." Then, they had to compete for openings. The combined degree evolved slowly into the current, much-strengthened five-year "medical/dental leadership program."

Public health was finally finding a place to stand in the sun.

A Crowning Achievement: The Preventive Medicine Residency

As already described, the story at Loma Linda goes back to the ideal of "medical missionary" work. In the 1920s, Dr. Newton Evans, then dean of the Los Angeles division of CME, bemoaned the lack of interest in public health at CME. Beyond interest, a lack of knowledge itself about public health prevailed. Referring back to the Church's early stand on "health reform," he noted that public health professional interest was moving from environmental sanitation to a large concern for personal hygiene and individual health promotion.

In 1928 the CME Board accepted a proposal from Evans. He had requested that a few selected fourth-year medical students be allowed to modify their senior year programs and continue on for an intern year in public health. Then, they would receive a "certificate of public health." Herein, Loma Linda made one of the first attempts anywhere to train physicians as public health specialists, certainly the first in the western United States. Eleven medical students enthusiastically signed up for the new program.

Then the National Board of Medical Examiners and the American Medical Association felled the proposal with a single blow. They refused to accept this new program in lieu of the regular required internship. This came despite endorsements from highly placed professors at Yale University and elsewhere. It would be twenty more years later (in 1948) before the American Board of Preventive Medicine was formed and finally approved public health/preventive medicine residency requirements.

In the meantime, back in Loma Linda the idea of a preventive medicine residency did not emerge again until in the 1960s. Dr. Elvin E. Adams, fresh from his MPH study at Johns Hopkins University, was accepted as the SPH's first post-doctoral fellow in preventive medicine (1969). Cheerful announcements of a forth-coming residency were made in 1970 and again in 1974. The actual launching, however, finally came in 1979, in a cooperative effort. The Schools of Public Health and Medicine now parented peacefully together and launched the new residency.

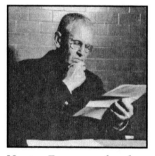

Newton Evans served as dean and as president of CME. In 1928 he formulated for CME one of the first plans for specialty training in public health in the world.

A preventive medicine residency is a substantial three-year plan that begins with a first year in any primary clinical specialty (commonly internal medicine or family medicine). The second year is devoted to the study for an MPH degree, with the third year spent in practical experience and research. At Loma Linda, the second and third years have always been tightly integrated, with the study and experience spread over both years.

The Support System

Several important local affiliations support Loma Linda's preventive medicine residency, providing both clinical experience and research opportunities. Loma Linda's residency is unique in the United States, and is the envy of many other preventive medicine residencies. Recognizing the benefit to them, all affiliations pay direct support to the residency and its budgets for residents.

This general preventive-medicine residency has been successfully operating now for more than 25 years. It operates under the department of preventive medicine in the School of Medicine. (Dr. Allan Darnell directs this residency in 2006.) In 2000, the acute shortage of occupational medicine professionals stimulated the beginning of that sub-specialty at Loma Linda.

The great news in January 2006 is that both the American Board of Family Medicine and the American Board of Preventive Medicine have approved Loma Linda's new sub-specialty in "lifestyle medicine." The first such program to be approved anywhere, this four-year program will include an MPH degree from the SPH and make graduates board-eligible in both specialties—family and preventive medicine. Most importantly, it will be the first medical training program specifically designed to train physicians to help prevent, treat, and provide long-term health maintenance. Those with such lifestyle disease problems as coronary atherosclerosis, diabetes, hypertension, obesity, and related lifestyle manifestations are the beneficiaries. These problems, of course, are now pandemic around the world.

The following local affiliations are very supportive and greatly appreciated in this Loma Linda preventive medicine training:

The LLU Center for Health Promotion. Services include weight management, smoking cessation, alcohol and drug recovery, executive health, physical fitness testing and counseling, and a travel clinic. This is one of the primary clinical settings for the residency.

The Jerry L. Pettis Memorial Veterans Administration Medical Center initiated its support of the residency in 1986, with P. William Dysinger as its first program director. The VA hospital currently supports five PM residents, more than twice as many as any other VA hospital in that large system.

Kaiser Permanente Medical Center, an HMO in Fontana, has provided excellent clinical experience in its Center for Health Promotion, as well as a good introduction to work in the HMO setting.

Patton State Hospital provides significant experience in administration and policy development and in disease surveillance.

San Bernardino County Health Department, the largest (in area) in the United States, provides a wide variety of public health experiences. The current health department director is a graduate of the Loma Linda residency and takes personal interest in all residents in their program.

The Inland Empire Health Plan is a MediCal HMO that also provides residents with a wide variety of general preventive medicine experiences as well as occupational medicine experience.

Chaffee, Riverside City, and San Bernardino Valley Colleges. LLU, under contract, provides student health services to more than 40,000 students enrolled in these community colleges. The residency also helps provide health services to students at both Redlands and Loma Linda universities.

Loma Linda University Medical Center provides funding for four residents, two in the intern clinical year, and two in second and/or third year positions.

The LLU School of Public Health has always been a strong supporter of the PM residency. It not only provides offices and an academic home for the residency, but also provides some tuition support. It otherwise provides special tracks in all departments for residents to complete their required MPH concurrently with their residency training.

The medical school d*epartment of family medicine* has joined with the department of preventive medicine to give an integrated program in "lifestyle medicine." This arrangement provides a unique blending of primary health care and preventive medicine.

A series of distinguished directors have brought preventive medicine at Loma Linda to its present state of prosperity. Its residency has been recognized as one of ten model programs among the more than 80 preventive-medicine residencies in North America. As of August 2003, 107 physicians have completed their PM residencies at Loma Linda. They now hold leadership positions all around the world.

Richard H. Hart was chair of preventive medicine for almost twenty years. After serving two years as chancellor of LLU, he turned responsibility for the department over to Wayne S. Dysinger in July 2003. (Wayne is the son of Dr. and Mrs. P. William Dysinger). Dr. Wayne Dysinger is boarded in both family medicine and preventive medicine and brings to Loma Linda his background of eleven years of experience in teaching these disciplines at the Georgia Baptist Hospital in Atlanta and at Dartmouth University in New Hampshire. He feels much encouraged about the prospects of preventive and lifestyle medicine at Loma Linda.

At long last, a very old Loma Linda dream is materializing.

27

The Disease Detectives

N owadays, the injunction "to publish or perish" prevails in all reputable universities. Every academic knows that he/she must heed that admonition or pay a costly, even embarrassing, price. For several reasons, the impetus to do productive research at Loma Linda developed slowly. With CME often fighting for its very survival, research seemed to be a luxury no one could afford. Still, the accrediting association, like a mother-in-law who visits too often, shadowed the University. Over time, this pressure became very palpable.

The desire to do research at CME, however, is traceable back at least to 1928. The medical faculty formed a research organization, at that time. They named it the "Harveian Society," in honor of the English anatomist, William Harvey (1578–1657), who discovered the circulation of the blood. From the start, they declared that CME's deficiency in research had not been "from any lack of individual scientific interest." Good as their word, they reported at least eight (internally funded) research projects the next year. They also expressed appreciation for the recently established research laboratory at Loma Linda.

The Harveian Society had very specific procedures. Every month each member had to present a typewritten abstract of two accomplishments: a practical subject for publication and a topic for discussion. For many years these summaries of disease problems featured regularly in *The Medical Evangelist*. Dean Edward H. Risley enthusiastically praised the research achievements of the Harveian Society.

In 1931 a research committee recommended prioritizing programs that would work upon problems "which would be definitely related to our special beliefs as a denomination." Safe as this proposal might be, no action was ever taken.

Dr. P. T. Magan, the president, also had very specific ideas (1933). The administrators, he said, struggled just "to keep the school going." Tuition money should be spent for the students rather than "highbrow researchers." Furthermore, those who "make good research workers, as a rule, are wretched schoolteachers." But "above all things" CME had to emphasize "as never before ... [its] medical-missionary and spiritual phases." These attitudes, of course, explain why the research efforts of the School of Medicine were so meager.

The admirable Harveian Society notwithstanding, some members of the American Medical Association criticized CME roundly. One pontificated: "It is the function of every medical school to teach and to do research, and, I may add, to care for the sick in its hospitals." Any teacher who "has not been bitten by the research bug," he said, "is not a real teacher." Forestalling any other possible excuses, he concluded, "There is so much that is unknown that it is not difficult to find a research problem" (1939).

The Quest for Grants

Obviously, research calls for money. A lot of it. One of the first externally funded research grants for Loma Linda came, appropriately, from the Review and Herald Publishing Association (1945). *Life and Health* was known to be "one of the most important means ... for carrying [our] health teachings to the world." Therefore, $25,000 from the magazine's earnings were set aside for the "Life and Health Research Foundation." Insofar as "these resources permit," investigations should be made in such areas as nutrition and physical therapy and reported in "a manner most likely to convince thoughtful men of their soundness."

CME received this boon as "a good thing." Apart from work in nutrition (see chapter 5), however, no records remain to tell us about any other research. Some of the Foundation funds were used to help found a scientific quarterly, *Medical Arts and Sciences*, published by the University. Its timing was propitious and its publication continued into the late 1970s.

A year later, Dr. Newton Evans formed the "Alumni Research Foundation." At the constituency meeting, however, the president apologized: "It is not our intention to spend too much time or money on research activities." As it turned out, the main purpose was simply "to obtain funds."

Out of this context comes the research story of the School of Tropical and Preventive Medicine (see chapter 7).

Nonetheless, voices doggedly pleading for more research rose on all sides. Dr. J. Dewitt Fox of White Memorial Hospital, for example, hoped that his cancer research would help put CME on the right road. Moreover, he realized that all of the faculty needed to be regularly informed about trends in American medical research.

By 1953 CME was one of fourteen medical education centers listed by *Science* magazine to have shown "the most rapid increase in research potentials." In 1950 Loma Linda ranked 17 places higher than it had in 1944. A somewhat "backhanded" compliment perhaps, considering the low level at its start. By 1959, however, activities had become quite commendable, partly due to the influence of Bruce Halstead and the old STPM. The School of Medicine now had 172 research projects under way, and 185 publications had been generated from this spurt of energy.

Enter Biostatistics

As the foundation of research and analysis, the study of statistics is essential. A physicist, Dr. Robert Woods, became the first statistician on Loma Linda's campus. He developed a course for the medical students and helped provide statistical planning for all university research projects.

The first fully qualified biostatistician at LLU, Jan Kuzma, arrived in 1963. He served the University for the next twenty-three years. He organized and chaired the SPH's department of biostatistics. In addition to his departmental responsibilities, Kuzma worked as an examiner in the Riverside Health Department. His first major grant ($114,400) came from NIH Institute of Alcohol Abuse and Alcoholism. As principal investigator, he studied the effects of alcohol and pregnancy, a hot topic in 1973. His research, in fact, helped define the very destructive fetal-alcohol syndrome. Then, drawing on his years of research

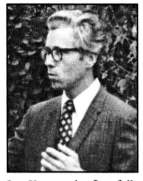

Jan Kuzma, the first fully qualified biostatistician at Loma Linda, served as first chair of the department of biostatistics and Loma Linda's first research director.

and teaching, Kuzma wrote a widely used textbook, *Basic Statistics for the Health Sciences*.

Also, the School of Public Health's department of biostatistics was a service unit for the entire University. By offering advanced computer programming, it provided the resources to solve practical public health problems. Consultation on research protocols and the evaluation of data came with the territory. Even though biostatistics aided many other disciplines, it never attracted many graduate students.

Initially carrying a nameless portfolio, Kuzma usually introduced himself as the "director of research at LLU School of Public Health." Out of his work, in the mid-1980s, grew the Center for Health Research (CHR).

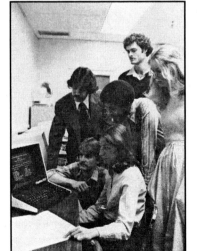

Students analyzing computer data for a research project.

It has become home base for encouraging and coordinating health research, especially in the School of Public Health.

Before Dr. Kuzma's retirement in 1990, other biostatisticians had come on board: Paul Y. Yahiku, Grennith Zimmerman, David Abbey, Robert J. Cruise, Gerald W. Shavlik, and others. Supplying the general need for basic biostatistics teaching in the University increased course offerings and provided research assistance as technology proliferated.

To cope with all of these burgeoning complexities, Dr. David Abbey introduced a new advantage to the University and to the public, the "Survey Research Service" (1973). SRS would conserve money for such concerns as coronary risk evaluation, the demographics of population, and many other kinds of health surveys. The organization designed questionnaires and collected, processed, and analyzed data. An early customer, the Environmental Protection Agency (EPA), wanted a study on the effects of air pollution on human health. By 1985 SRS was pulling in significant income from its enormous variety and range of clients.

Although now retired, Abbey remains an important survey specialist for Loma Linda University.

The Ultimate Investigators

Epidemiology is the "intelligence service" for all health programs. First, it searches out the origins of disease and clarifies the risk factors. Then it examines the importance of environment, human biology (including genetics), and lifestyle on the prevalence of disease. It also measures how organized health care systems relate to the state of people's health and seeks to quantify health.

Epidemiology is a basic discipline taught to all medical and health science students. Loma Linda has utilized these detective skills to research the significant differences between Seventh-day Adventists and the general population in regard to morbidity (illness data), mortality, and life expectancy. These discoveries attracted much media attention in 2005 after *National Geographic* magazine featured Loma Linda and Adventists in a cover story on longevity.

As CME's first epidemiologist, Dr. Frank R. Lemon, along with Dr. Richard T. Walden, organized the first Adventist Mortality Study (AMS). After being

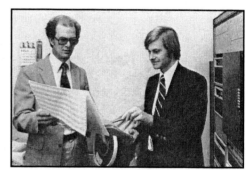

Roland Phillips (left) and Gary Fraser (right), important leaders of the Adventist Health Studies. Phillips initiated the studies and Fraser is the current director.

independent during their first years of organization, biostatistics and epidemiology joined together to form the department of epidemiology and biostatistics. Epidemiology, in particular, continued to multiply, attracting grants from many sources. Much could be said of Loma Linda's epidemiologists. Among them would be Dr. Raymond O. West who has, for many years, taught basic epidemiology both on and off campus. Other distinguished professors have followed.

Roland L. Phillips was the first doctoral-trained (Johns Hopkins University) epidemiologist on campus and he initiated the NCI funded Adventist Health Study. He had a passion for research, rather than administration or academics. He had recognition nationwide as one of the foremost investigators in cancer and lifestyle medicine. Unfortunately, at the peak of an outstanding career, he died in a sailplane accident in 1987.

Gary Fraser from New Zealand capably replaced Phillips. With help from a $305,000 grant he was able to produce his well-known textbook, *Preventive Cardiology* (Oxford Press 1986). Then, with two more NIH grants, he was able to add a new heart disease component to the Adventist Heath Studies, followed by $1 million for a study on aging. Next, after three years' effort, Fraser secured $18 million to further expand yet another Adventist Health Study.

Following his years at Loma Linda, David Snowden pursued the exciting work of directing "The Nuns' Study" (1984). Holding appointments in both epidemiology and preventive medicine, he and Paul K. Mills managed "damage control." The Adventist Health Study came under scrutiny because of the largely Adventist staff. "Surely, they would put their personal bias into the study and skew its results." Because neither Snowden nor Mills were Adventists, their good work did much to increase the credibility of the study. Actually, this wasn't really necessary; the Adventist investigators bent over backwards to guarantee that their studies and reports would be unbiased.

The current chair of LLU's very active combined department of epidemiology and biostatistics, Dr. Synnove Knutsen, has worked with several large EPA-funded studies Although a "young" discipline, epidemiology has always been a lively program at the School of Public Health, at both the doctoral and masters levels. Loma Linda's epidemiology graduates continue to be in demand and occupy important positions around the world.

The Adventist Advantage

Today no one argues against the idea that lifestyle choices make a tremendous difference to the quality of life. The Adventist Health Studies (AHS) have been a long-standing work-in-progress. Over the past 45 years private foundations and the United States government have invested more than $40 million dollars in this Loma Linda enterprise. Dr. Walter Willets, chair of the department of nutrition in the Harvard School of Public Health, said: "Long term studies like the Adventist study are really the only way we can fully understand how diet will impact our health … [and] how we can reduce our risk of cancer." An eminent Stanford epidemiologist, Ralph Paffenberger, added, "Adventists are a national treasure for health research."

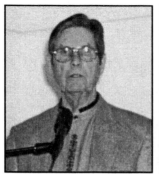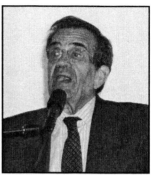

Frank Lemon (left) and Ernst Wynder (right) initiated the first studies where Seventh-day Adventists were named. There are now more than 300 published study reports of Seventh-day Adventists—the most researched religious group in history.

Several findings emerging out of LLU's School of 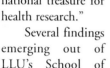 Public Health Adventist Health Studies have, indeed, become familiar in the public arena. Even commonplace. For example, "Eat more fruits and vegetables, at least five servings a day." Other findings: eating whole wheat bread can reduce the risk of non-fatal heart attacks by 45 percent; persons eating nuts five or more times a week have a 50 percent less risk of heart attack than those who do not; a high consumption of tomatoes can reduce men's risk of prostate cancer by 40 percent; also, drinking five or more glasses of water daily may reduce the risk of heart attack by 50 percent.

Ironically, when Mervyn Hardinge proposed the first study of Adventist vegetarians for his Harvard doctoral dissertation, his Loma Linda advisors vetoed his plan. "You will have to change your research project."

"But why?" Hardinge wanted to know.

"Because if you find that the diets of vegetarians are deficient, it will embarrass us."

"Well," Hardinge reasoned, "if the diets are inadequate, we should be the first to find out. We shouldn't leave it up to others." He won his point.

When he completed his DrPH (1951), the *Journal of the American Dietetic Association* published his research in a series of five articles: "Nutritional Studies of Vegetarians." This history-making work appeared under the names of Hardinge and his advisor, Frederick J. Stare, the chair of the nutrition department at Harvard. No one mentioned, however, that this was a study of Adventists.

In the 1950s Dr. Ernest Wynder, an epidemiologist with the Sloan-Kettering Memorial Cancer Institute of New York, was trying to confirm the connections between cigarette smoking and cancer and cardio-vascular disease. Because Adventists offered him the non-smoking population group he needed, he ended up working with Dr. Frank Lemon at White Memorial Hospital in Los Angeles. His report documenting much less cancer and heart disease in Adventists not only stimulated further research, but it also was the first peer-reviewed scientific article to mention Seventh-day Adventists by name (1959). Today well over 300 such articles exist.

A Triple Achievement in the School of Public Health
In the past 50 years three major studies have taken place at Loma Linda.

1. The Adventist Mortality Study (AMS, 1955–1975) by Drs. Frank Lemon and Richard Walden was the first epidemiologic prospective study of Adventists. It began with a three-year study of lung and laryngeal cancer, funded by an NIH grant of $73,500. Next, the Nutritional Foundation in New York released another grant for a companion study: "The Dietary, Environmental, and Cultural Factors in Coronary Artery Disease." Meticulously, Lemon and Walden canvassed the 65,000 Adventists in California. The initial, simple enrollment form was followed by a registration questionnaire. They confined the study to the "actual available" church members, particularly those over the age of twenty-nine.

The registration questionnaire was identical to that used by the American Cancer Society. Therefore, the Adventists could readily be compared with the one million people of the general population already in the ACS files. The death records, gleaned from many sources, told a very cheerful story about the health of Adventists! For good reason, the School of Public Health conferred its Distinguished Service Award on Lemon and Walden in 1998.

2. The Adventist Health Study I (AHS-1, 1975–2002) enrolled a second cohort of Adventists in California (persons over twenty-five years of age) and studied their health data. This time, the survey included some Hispanics and Blacks. Nutrition was especially emphasized in this study. Enrollees answered 55 food-frequency questions, as well as a dozen other dietary inquiries. The validation of the unique food-frequency surveys became a very important addition to the study. The investigators followed all subjects for six years in order to collect all new cases of cancer and coronary heart disease.

3. The Adventist Health Study II (AHS-2, 2002–the present) has become "bigger and better" than any of its predecessors. It intends to enroll 125,000 Adventists (from 4,300 churches) across all of North America. With these large numbers, minimal differences in lifestyle can become statistically significant in health outcomes and disease or death. Hopefully, participants will be tracked for twenty years, with updates every five years. All of this activity requires a staff of more than 50 researchers to manage this large population as well as all the collected data.

The results of the Adventist Health Studies have now been published in more than 320 peer-reviewed scientific articles in the most important science or medical journals in the world. The conclusions have been enough to stop traffic all over the earth. California Adventist vegetarians live substantially longer than other Californians, an average of 9.5 years for males (6.2 years for females). Not only do they live longer, but Adventist vegetarians also have a better quality of life (at any age). With less cancer, heart disease, diabetes, arthritis, and hypertension, they use health services less frequently and take fewer medications than non-vegetarian Adventists.

Seventh-day Adventists have been formally identified and described as the longest-lived population group in California. Indeed, they have been made a "spectacle to the world, both to angels and to men" (I Corinthians 4:9). Many people, both on and off campus, are interested in this mix of research results at Loma Linda.

28

A Newcomer with an Ancient Past

From ancient times many people have practiced cleanliness and personal hygiene, often for religious reasons. The Mosaic Laws in Old Testament scripture comprise one of the earliest sanitation codes we have on record. The Hebrews carefully differentiated clean and unclean living and foods. The Greeks developed the idea that pestilence might come from natural causes. Hippocrates (born 460 BC) wrote *Airs, Waters, and Places*, a treatise that, for more than 2,200 years, provided the theoretical basis for understanding endemic diseases. Given the antiquity of the book, of course, it contained some misinformation. For instance, Hippocrates knew that malaria (literally "bad air") was connected with swamps. The knowledge of the mosquito as the villain came many centuries later. Although the new ideas were accepted slowly, every graduating physician today very properly takes the Oath of Hippocrates, truly the "Father of Medicine."

Through the centuries a devastating procession of epidemics and pestilences have scarred the world populations. In the mid-fourteenth century, the Black Death surged out of Central Asia to be carried on ships to Constantinople, Genoa, and other European ports. This dramatic sequence of events spread the disease to the interior, killing at least twenty-five million in Europe alone. Since the plague was connected to ships, ports like Venice and Marseilles adopted a 40-day quarantine period. For the first time, governments established the *cordon sanitaire* and took a hand in disease control.

The grim "mortality lists" (statistics) caused anguish and panic as people faced the dreaded epidemic diseases like plague, yellow fever, smallpox, and cholera. As a result, four basic public health activities became the foundation of public health: 1) environmental sanitation, 2) medical care of the poor, 3) quarantine, and 4) the control of communicable diseases.

Just prior to the founding of Loma Linda, several important 19th-century discoveries paved the way in the practice of environmental health. An Italian bacteriologist, Agostino Bassi (1773–1856), dealing with silkworm infections, found that a number of diseases were caused by specific organisms. The French chemist Louis Pasteur (1822–1895) and the German Robert Koch (1843–1910) developed methods for isolating and characterizing bacteria and relating them to specific diseases such as tuberculosis. A Nobel Prize-winning English physician Sir Ronald Ross (1857–1932) identified the mosquito as the carrier of malaria. The French epidemiologist Paul-Louis Simond (1858–1937) produced evidence to show that the plague was primarily a disease of rats. Two Americans, Walter Reed (1851–1902) and James Carroll demonstrated that yellow fever came from a virus carried by mosquitoes.

To put the above achievements in perspective, we look at a statement in CME's *The Medical Evangelist*, July 12, 1923, which indicates how recent these findings were: "Ninety years ago today there was not a single disease afflicting the human race, the cause of which was known."

At the turn of the 20th century, health departments tried hard to improve environmental conditions, sanitation and general hygiene. Bacteriologists identified disease-causing microorganisms: leprosy (1873); typhoid (1880); malaria (1880); tuberculosis (1882); diphtheria (1883); cholera (1884); tetanus (1884); and plague (1894). With this knowledge, new specific vaccines could be prepared to combat these terrors.

The effects of these controls brought about another happy circumstance. Infant and child mortality dropped sharply, and life expectancy increased measurably. By 2000, deaths from infectious ailments had markedly declined. Degenerative diseases associated with aging, however, rapidly replaced them.

"Environment" is defined as "the surroundings, conditions, or influences that affect an organism." Besides water purification and improved sanitation, LLU reckoned in five other environmental interventions: 1) control of disease carrying insects or animals, 2) adequately ventilated housing, 3) reduction of occupational/industrial risks, 4) reduction of air and water pollution, and 5) safety, including the control of road traffic and impaired driving.

Environmental Health at Loma Linda

At the beginning of the College of Evangelists we detect only minimal interest in environmental health. In the first academic bulletin no such course appears. A half unit in "bacteriology," however, did show up. Then the importance of this study increased dramatically over the next nine years. By 1915 the bacteriology course had leaped to 50 lecture hours plus 110 laboratory hours. In 1919 the Board of Trustees even empowered CME to spend $2,000 on the "prevention of flies and mosquitoes," in order to deal with local problems.

Shortly after the founding of the School of Public Health, Dr. Elmer A. Widmer, joined the faculty (1967). As a parasitologist with a special interest in ecology, he became the first chair of the department of environmental health. He quickly involved the School in community projects. For instance, Loma Linda faculty joined State Assemblyman Biddle's air pollution advisory committee and the new environmental protection commission in Riverside, California. This community was one of the first United

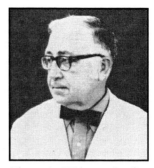

Elmer A. Widmer, the first chair of environmental health at Loma Linda.

States cities to concern itself with saving the environment. Certified as a diplomate of the American Academy of Sanitarians (1988), Widmer served the ENVH department continuously for twenty-one years.

Karl Fischer taught a course, "tropical housing and sanitation" (1970). His students came to Loma Linda from Ghana, Ethiopia, the Congo, Thailand, and Singapore. Then Robert F. Wood, a sanitary engineer, helped publicize the SPH with his research in water pollution control. Dr. Albert Whiting, Franklin Crider, and Alan R. Magie all served in the department of environmental and tropical health. During his chairmanship Magie reorganized the department to provide three majors: environmental health, parasitology, and tropical health. In 1972 he landed a five-year-grant of $179,824 to provide training for environmentalists. With a later grant he went on to investigate the effects of smog on the health of college students.

The next departmental re-organization (1982) revealed that LLU was moving away from tropical health toward other concerns. From a new interest in "occupational environment," four areas of emphasis emerged: environmental health, environmental health management, human ecology, and industrial hygiene. Soon after, the department dropped "tropical" from its name.

A couple of interesting stories came out of LLU's experiments in environmentalism. David Specht, one of Widmer's graduate students, discovered asexual reproduction in the Mexocestoides tapeworm (1963). Forthwith, the humble tapeworm ascended to the position of being a very valuable research subject in biology and medicine. In 1987, Frederick D. Schmidt (an ENVH graduate) worked for the California Air Resources Board. He proudly showed to his alma mater the only mobile fuel-toxics laboratory existing at the time.

When Dr. George Johnston became ENVH program director, he added "toxic risk assessment" to the MSPH menu (1990). All of this called for yet another name-change, "department of environmental and occupational health."

179

A New Look in an Old Department (1992–2004)

With the coming of David and Angela Dyjack (a SPH graduate), environmentalism at Loma Linda got a new boost (1992). She was a graduate of the School of Public Health. The Dyjacks had established themselves as environmental health consultants in Washington, D.C.

Upon joining the SPH faculty, they combined their industrial health expertise with the already-existing momentum in environmental health. The new dimension in occupational health was strengthened. Even before they graduated, many Loma Linda environmental students found employment with the EPA, the United States Department of Energy, Exxon, Texaco, Mobil, Disney, and other companies.

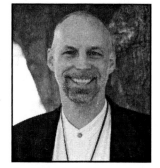

A CEPH accreditation visit in 1993 had had positive outcomes. The only question raised? A concern that the department of environmental and occupational health "lacked senior leadership." Two years later this thinly veiled reference to the necessity of the almighty doctorate resulted in a $20,000 grant from Ford Motor Company to help fund David Dyjack's completion of his DrPH research.

David Dyjack pioneered the degree program in public health practice. He has been very active in applied programs in public health.

At the same time, he easily stayed in contact with the "real world." Dyjack became a consulting compliance officer for California OSHA. The regional manager of OSHA said, "We always have more inspections to make and accidents to investigate than we have people to take care of them." Dyjack's consultancy services served them well, and he presented several seminars on indoor air quality—one in Seoul, Korea.

Dr. Padma P. Uppala, an environmental toxicologist, opened up a new field of study at Loma Linda. By investigating the human genome and its relation to disease, she became a leader in genomics research. With a $250,000 grant in 2003, she began examining the protective effect of certain foods against breast cancer. Thus, she held out a ray of hope for those predisposed to that killer disease. At this same time, the SPH environmental health department began to partner with the United States Peace Corps International.

In this new millennium the department of environmental and occupational health has attained a solid track record. One that has attracted several federal grants. Loma Linda is one of four schools of public health in California that make up a consortium called "The Pacific Public Health Training Center." LLU's contributions include a multi-lingual CD-ROM that instructs county health employees in the core functions and essential services of public health. Within this consortium Loma Linda is also involved in training in food-borne illness, risk communication, environmental disparities, and asthma triggers.

In 2004 the United States Centers for Disease Control and Prevention funded the Loma Linda School of Public Health as an eight-state environmental health resource center for Native Americans. Many of the tribes lack the technical expertise to look after their own health. Here Loma Linda steps in, as requested, with technical advice.

Having a well-qualified faculty, the department receives a steady flow of grants, as it actively reflects the rapidly changing world around it. Therefore, the future looks bright.

One More Unique Touch

As the SPH developed its international health program in 1967, Dr. Robert Cleveland, (LLU vice president for academic affairs) introduced a unique element into the mix. The relationships between population densities, climate, altitude, vegetation and food supplies, industrialization, and many other environmental situations interested him. As a geographer, he inaugurated Loma Linda's early collection of non-political maps. It became the largest map collection of its kind in Southern California, and was well used, at that time, by many public health teachers.

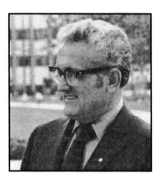

More recently, mapping has become computerized. Housed in the department of environmental and occupational health, this practical new technology is called "geographic information systems" (GIS). It has opened up crucial new areas of investigation at Loma Linda. The eighteen-seat geoinformatics unit laboratory provides state-of-the-art facilities for GIS training and research. Situated on campus in the Del E. Webb Memorial Library, it is the first lab of its kind in the United States. At the same time, it is the physical home for the first public health GIS certificate (health geoinformatics) offered in the world.

Robert Cleveland, as vice president for academic affairs, assisted the SPH in collecting the largest environmental, non-political map collection in Southern California.

The lab is an outstanding research tool in epidemiologic and other spatial studies. It is well used by the Seventh-day Adventist Church as well as many other private and public entities.

29

What's So Important About Health?

Modern organizations and public health workers go to great lengths to prevent unnecessary disease and to preserve "complete physical and mental well-being." Even so, good health is not a commercial commodity. At least 70 percent of optimum health comes from a person's own lifestyle choices.

What's important about health? Even after all of the evidence is in, the casual reader may still be asking this question. Many, including some quite notable people, have personally discovered the answer.

A 180-Degree Turn

Early in life John Davison Rockefeller, Sr. (1839–1937) set himself the goal of earning money. A lot of it. To do so, he pushed himself to the limit. At 33, he had earned his first million dollars. By age 43, he controlled Standard Oil (Exxon), the largest company in the world, one that would dominate the oil industry for the next 40 years. At age 53, he was the world's richest man—the only billionaire at the time. He didn't have to do one thing further to earn his weekly income of more than $1 million.

By this time, however, Rockefeller had become physically ill, losing both his hair and weight. While hair loss is the plight of many men, a steady decline in weight certainly is not. This poor rich man couldn't sleep or enjoy much of anything in life. The only food he could eat and digest was milk and crackers. "You'll be fortunate," his physicians told him, 'if you can stay alive one more year."

One sleepless night Rockefeller came face to face with his own mortality. "Here I am, only 54 years old. All this money, and I can't take a penny of it to the next world." He realized that his money was worthless to buy back the health he had destroyed.

The next morning he got out of bed a new man.

A devout Baptist, he had, as a young man, paid tithe on his very first paycheck and had continued to do so. Now he went far beyond the routine kind of charitable donations. Plunging into an unbelievable amount of philanthropy, he began giving away his wealth, left, right, and center. His "Rockefeller Foundation" funded health care for people all over the world, initiating many good programs that still continue.

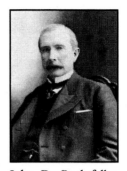

John D. Rockefeller, Sr., the world's first billionaire, almost died before he recognized the health benefits of good use of his money in helping others.

This charitable attitude now came back to heal him, both spiritually and physically. Immediately he began sleeping well, eating well, and, above all, finding meaning in life. This benevolent tycoon is said to have given a shiny dime to every child he met.

By changing his work habits and philosophy, JDR lived to a great old age, dying just two years short of his 100th birthday—a goal that he had set for himself at the time of his "conversion."

The Last Major Component of Good Health

Most people tend not to value health until they begin to lose it. After they have adopted all of the physical "rules of health," however, one vital element still remains, the spiritual. The ultimate enjoyment of good health depends on it, absolutely.

This essential additive to good health practices can be comprehended only in light of the "Great Controversy" between Christ and Satan. In the beginning God created man in His likeness, with the ability to grow and develop his every capability—physical, mental, and spiritual. Life had but one purpose—to live to bless others and thus glorify God and return love to Him.

Satan originated selfishness and self-seeking. In the Garden of Eden he caused Adam and Eve to doubt God and His goodness—His justice and terrible majesty. Satan further persuaded humankind to look upon God as severe and unforgiving. How could this misrepresentation be overcome? Only Christ, coming out of the glory of heaven itself, could demonstrate God's love. Nothing but the plan of salvation and the revelation of God in the life and death of Jesus on earth could answer the question, "Is God good?"

Sin, however, has marred and almost completely obliterated the image of God in man. In order to restore what had been lost, God gave humankind a life of "probation" on earth. Thus the great purpose of life here is to bring us back towards our original perfection. This objective underlies all others.

God's love, and His laws, reflect His character. Firstly, He has revealed himself to us in His Word. Secondly, we learn that human life is controlled by His immutable laws of nature. Since God has authored both, to transgress His physical laws is also to break His moral law. Misuse of physical powers, for example, shortens life and thus violates the sixth commandment against killing. God's love cannot be forced, however, so the final decision is left with us. In every case the selfish heart always lives to itself.

Will-power and Self-control

"The brain is the seat of our soul, will, and intellect. It is God's temple in which He desires to dwell" (1 Corinthians 3:16, 17; 6:19, 20). Anything that diminishes physical strength tends to weaken the mind, making it less capable of discriminating between right and wrong. How then can we choose the good and have the will-power to do what we know to be right?

As a matter of fact, most people know how to live better than they do. Those who don't know need to be taught. The majority just need to understand the importance of their daily life choices. In other words, we can learn the lifestyle of heaven while here on earth. Healthy living, then, has great spiritual significance, teaching us how to better understand our relationship with God. The bottom line, as John D. Rockefeller learned, is that philanthropy and medical missionary endeavor cures selfishness, directly promotes health, and proves God is good.

Loma Linda, Flagship of Health Reform

How much one can earn health by keeping nature's laws has definite limits. God's healing power takes us beyond our keeping of His commands that prevent disease (Exodus 15:26).

On the other hand, God would hear the prayers of the sick among us more fully if people were not violating the laws of health by their personal choice. Finding relief from sickness by right habits of living and learning how to avoid sickness must be our goal. "The sincerity of our prayers can be proved only by the vigor of our endeavor to obey God's commandments."

Two weeks after its organization (1863) God gave the Seventh-day Adventist Church a distinctive health message. This, Ellen White's first vision after the formal organization of the Seventh-day Adventist Church, clarified God's wish to be glorified by the life and health of His people. A comprehensive health message has been beautifully delineated in her book *Ministry of Healing*. Much research at Loma Linda and elsewhere has now confirmed well these principles.

A Patient's Obligation

The body is the only medium through which the mind and the soul can build character (*Ministry of Healing*). Our tools, will and self-control, must be used daily as we choose food or drink, find the balance between exercise and rest, and practice other elements of lifestyle. Consequently, these small choices of daily life provide an excellent field for character development. Only by the grace of God can any of us find such self-control—and sanctification. Paul announced: "I can do everything through Him who gives me strength" (Philippians 4:13).

We have a clear mission. We must nurture completely trustworthy people who understand that disobeying God's laws, physical or moral, leads to disease and death. God's way, on the other hand, leads us into life and health, and—at last—into Eternity. "One of the most deplorable effects of the original apostasy (in Eden) was the loss of man's power of self-control. Only as this power is regained, can there be real progress." Beyond feelings and theory, true "sanctification" is a "living, active principle, entering into the everyday life." Our habits of "eating, drinking, and dressing" contribute to the preservation of "physical, mental, and moral health" (*Ministry of Healing*).

The Apostle Paul skillfully summed up this imperative: "Everyone who competes in the games (of life) goes into strict training. They (athletes) do it to get a crown that will not last; but we do it to get a crown that will last forever. Therefore, I do not run like a man running aimlessly; I do not fight like a man beating the air. No, I beat my body and make it my slave so that after I have preached to others, I myself will not be disqualified for the prize" (1 Corinthians 9:25–27).

Balancing Faith and Works

Study of our human bodies and our health practices teaches us that God expects a balance between faith and works. We must avoid the belief that we can earn health by our own effort alone. At the other extreme, we cannot expect a miracle of God's healing simply because He loves us. Or that He will heal us, no matter what our lifestyle. Humans have a hard time accepting the balance between faith and works (James 2:17). Our highest motivation for living a healthy lifestyle should be the desire to reveal God in our bodies, our words, and our actions. Our willingness to fully reveal God in this way becomes our grateful tribute to Him.

We can "patiently endure" because of Christ's victory. By placing our will totally in His hands, we too may have the victory. "It is God who works in you to will and to act according to His good purpose" (Philippians 2:13). Moreover, He "is able to do immeasurably more than all we ask or imagine, according to His power that is at work within us, to Him be glory in the church" (Ephesians 3:20, 21). Not our power, but His. Our part is to invite Him into our lives and allow Him to work through us.

Challenge to Christian Health Workers

Ever since the Seventh-day Adventist Church established CME 100 years ago, faculty and students have been studying ways to encourage and keep people healthy. The Adventist Health Studies have clearly documented the Adventist health advantage. One SPH graduate, David Nieman, however, points out a paradox: "It is curious that so many Seventh-day Adventists have not made the decision to fully enter into this [now well-established] lifestyle."

In an interesting way, ancient Israel's travel from Egypt to the "Promised Land" parallels the preparation we need today. "Now all these things happened to them [Israel] as examples, and they were written for our admonition, upon whom the ends of the ages have come" (1 Corinthians 10:11).

Consider the first pledge given to Israel after they crossed the Red Sea en route to their Promised Land: "If you diligently heed the voice of the Lord your God and do what is right in His sight, give ear to His commandments and keep all His statutes, I will put none of the diseases on you which I have brought on the Egyptians. For I am the Lord who heals you" (Exodus 15:26). This, indeed, was a health message! It called for specific diet reform, health rules, and observance of the laws of sanitation and hygiene.

In the last days of earth's history, we are told that "the creation eagerly waits for the revealing of the sons of God," who are designated to be "a spectacle to the world" (Romans 8:19; 1 Corinthians 4:9). Today, more than 320 reports in the scientific literature have indeed made Seventh-day Adventists a "spectacle." Never before have scientists given this much attention to a religious group.

Despite their waywardness and disobedience, "[God] brought [Israel] out with silver and gold, and there was none feeble among His tribes." Why did God give them health? "That they might observe His statutes and keep His laws. Praise the Lord!" (Psalms 105:37, 45).

A Serious Responsibility

Many Seventh-day Adventists (even students and faculty at Loma Linda) have failed to live up to the health messages given to the Church—and specifically to Loma Linda. Still, God has been merciful, and the Adventist health studies document significantly better health in the study subjects than in the general population. Indeed, this finding has proven true in every country where Adventist health studies have been conducted.

"Behold what manner of love the Father has bestowed on us, that we should be called children of God …. It has not yet been revealed what we shall be, but we know that when He is revealed, we shall be like Him, for we shall see Him as He is. And everyone who has this hope in Him purifies himself, just as He is pure" (1 John 3:1-3).

The LLU School of Public Health can look to the future with hope. All of its disciplines have now become well established and have gained respect around the world. Because of the great need, however, we must build better organization and find more ways to "keep man whole." Above all, I believe the recognition of the spiritual significance of health is a tool that needs sharpening. We meet people where they are, and then go on to implant in them the highest motivation possible.

Harold Shull, an early health education professor in the School of Public Health, remembers a series of lectures given by Elder J. H. N. Tindall in the old STPM building (1965–1966, see chapter 2). This event occurred not long before Tindall died. The old man clearly remembered hearing Ellen White describe those who would be trained "on this Hill." They would proclaim the health reform message, she said, pointing to the spot where Nichol Hall now stands. Solemnly challenging the embryonic public health faculty, Tindall declared: "To this day, much that E. G. White described would take place on that hill has not been accomplished." Addressing the young professors, he added, "I challenge you to take up the gauntlet and, with much study and prayer, do the work that has not been and needs to be done."

A Tree of Life

For most of its history, the American Public Health Association had as its symbol a tree in a circle with the words, "And the leaves of the tree were for the healing of the nations" (Revelations 22:2). For a century now, Loma Linda has been identifying its own "health promoting leaves" to share with the world.

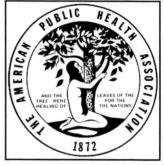

God has, indeed, blessed the School's efforts. What would be accomplished, however, if Loma Linda University and its School of Public Health, through study and prayer, could learn from the mistakes in its 100-year history? Can the School of Public Health become more successful in helping the public understand the spiritual significance of health and the God-created "Tree of Life?" Those leaves will permanently heal and preserve abundant health both in this life and in the eternal life to follow.

The American Public Health Association for much of its history used as its logo the "tree of life" shown here.

Many years ago, the American Public Health Association abandoned the tree-of-life motif as the symbol for the association. May Loma Linda never reject its spiritual heritage, its own "Tree of Life." May it understand and lovingly add the word "spiritual" to the World Health Organization definition of health "as complete physical, mental, and social well-being." No other institution can provide the world with what it needs as well as Loma Linda.

God will bless all who accept the challenge to take "health to the people" everywhere. And to take it in its most complete form.

Appendices

Appendix I

Glossary of Abbreviations and Terms Used

ACS	American Cancer Society
ADA	American Dietetics Association
ADRA	Adventist Development and Relief Agency (formerly SAWS)
AFB	Air Force Base
AHA	American Heart Association
AHI	Adventist Health International—an LLU consultative/training agency
AHS	Adventist Health Study or Adventist Health System, e.g. AHS/LL
AMA	American Medical Association (JAMA is Journal of AMA)
APHA	American Public Health Association
ASPH	Association of Schools of Public Health
AU	Andrews University, Berrien Springs, Michigan, U.S.A.
CAS	College of Arts and Sciences, La Sierra
CC	Conditioning Center—a lifestyle change facility
CDC	Centers for Disease Control and Prevention—Federal Agency in Atlanta
CE	Continuing Education
CEDB or CDB	The Center for Dependency Behavior
CEPH	Council on Education for Public Health—accrediting organization for PH
CHP	Center for Health Promotion—located in Evans Hall on LL campus
CHR	Center for Health Research, in the SPH
CME	The College of Medical Evangelists (at Loma Linda and in Los Angeles)
DDS	Doctor of dental surgery degree
DHSc	Doctor of health science degree (sometimes DrHSc or DHS is used)
DPH	Division of public health of the GS—direct predecessor to SPH, '64–'67
DPH&PM	Department of public health and preventive medicine of SM
DPH&TM	GS division of public health and tropical medicine (formerly STPM)
DPM	Department of preventive medicine of the SM
DPM&PH	Department of preventive medicine and public health of SM
DrPH	Doctor of public health degree—professional doctoral degree in PH
ENVH	Environmental health (LLU SPH department)
ENVH/OCCH	Environmental and occupational health (LLU SPH department)
ENVH/TROP	Environmental and tropical health (LLU SPH department)
EPA	Environmental Protection Agency (of the United States Government)
EPDM	Epidemiology (LLU SPH department)
EPDM/STAT	Epidemiology and biostatistics (LLU SPH department)

FHS	Family health services
FSI	Foreign Service Institute (training unit for the U.S. State Department)
GC	General Conference of Seventh-day Adventists (in Silver Spring, Maryland)
GIS	Geographic (or Global) information system—satellite mapping tool
GLOBHLTH	Global health (formerly international health) of LLU SPH
GS	Graduate School (after 1961) or School of Graduate Studies (before '61)
HADM	Health administration (LLU SPH department)
HADM/FHSE	Health administration and family health services (LLU department)
HLED	Health education (LLU SPH department)
HLSC	Health sciences, originally called health sciences and services
HPRO/EDUC	Health promotion and education (LLU SPH department)
ICPA	International Committee for the Prevention of Alcoholism
INTH	International health (LLU SPH department)
JLPMVH	Jerry L. Pettis Memorial Veterans Hospital (VA hospital in Loma Linda)
KCMC	Kilimanjaro Christian Medical Center near Moshi, Tanzania
LA	Los Angeles
LACH	Los Angeles County Hospital
LACHD	Los Angeles County Health Department
LIGA	Liga Mexico-PanAmerican Medico y Educacional, humanitarian aid agency
LL	Loma Linda
LLSH	Loma Linda Sanitarium and Hospital (now is Nichol Hall)
LLU	Loma Linda University
LLUMC	Loma Linda University Medical Center (the successor to the LLSH)
LLUAHSC	Loma Linda University Adventist Health Sciences Center
LSC	La Sierra College, Riverside (now Las Sierra University)
MC	Medical Center
MCH	Maternal (Mother) and child health
MD	Doctor of Medicine degree—the medical degree offered in the United States
MDiv	Master of divinity degree, the professional degree for ministers
ME	Medical evangelism, medical evangelistic or medical evangelist
MHA	Master of health administration degree
MIP	Master's international program (of the Peace Corps)
MM	Medical missionary
MPH	Master of public health (degree)—the qualifying degree in public health
MS	Master of science degree or Medical School
MSPH	Master of science in public health degree
NCI	National Cancer Institute (an NIH Institute)
NUTR	Nutrition (department), LLU, SPH
OSHA	Occupational Safety and Health Administration–United States Government agency
PASC	Pakistan Adventist Seminary and College—in the Punjab near Lahore
PH	Public health
PHC	Primary Health Care—a medical care movement that started in Alma Ata
PHPR	Public health practice
PHS	United States Public Health Service (also US PHS)
PM	Preventive medicine

PR	Public relations
PRVC	Preventive care
RCHD	Riverside County Health Department
RD	Registered dietitian
SAC	Social Action Corps
SAHP	School of Allied Health Professions, LLU
SAWS	Seventh-day World Service (now called ADRA)
SB	San Bernardino (city or county)
SBCH	San Bernardino County Hospital
SBCHD	San Bernardino County Health Department (or Dept. of PH)
SD	School of Dentistry
SH	School of Health—the name used by the SPH between 1970 and 1987
SIMS	Students for International Mission Service (originally "Medical Service")
SPH	School of Public Health
STAT	Biostatistics (department in the LLU SPH)
STPM	School of Tropical and Preventive Medicine of CME—1946–1960
TM	Tropical medicine
TRPH	Tropical health or tropical public health (LLU department or program)
UCLA	University of California, Los Angeles
USAID	United States Agency for International Development, the foreign aid branch of the United States Department of State
USPHS	United States Public Health Service
WASC	Western Association of Schools and Colleges (general accrediting association)
WCTU	Women's Christian Temperance Union
WHO	The World Health Organization (of the United Nations—is in Geneva)
WMH	White Memorial Hospital (located in East Los Angeles)
WMMC	White Memorial Medical Center—the current designation for the former WMH

Appendix II

A Selective Loma Linda Public Health Chronology

1. **May 26, 1905.** Purchase of original Loma Linda property by J. H. Burden.
2. **October 4, 1906.** Loma Linda College of Evangelists convened, starting with the nurse training program and the three-year-training course for "evangelistic-medical" (medical evangelistic) students (the first public health education effort at Loma Linda).
3. **November 29, 1908.** Farewell reception for Miss Meda Kerr, first Loma Linda graduate (a nurse medical-evangelist) to enter foreign mission service (served in Argentina, South America).
4. **September 1909.** "Cooks and bakers" course began. Offered as an annual nine-month course (until 1918).
5. **February 27, 1910.** Ellen G. White's "medical evangelism" vision.
6. **September 29, 1910.** CME medical school opened. Ten students, almost all transferred from medical evangelistic program.
7. **October 22, 1913.** Report to Board: "Schools of Health" demonstrated to be good means of increasing Sanitarium patronage. Voted to continue them.
8. **August 17, 1915.** Announcement: Faculty arranged a two-year "didactic and practical course" for medical evangelism students. Program opened in September, 39 students enrolled.
9. **April 21, 1920.** Board voted: Medical-evangelistic course be shortened to 12 months.
10. **September 10, 1922.** New "Dietitian's Training School," initiated by Harold M. Walton (first male dietitian with active membership in the American Dietetic Association, chartered 1917). New one-year medical missionary course instituted at same time.
11. **September 28, 1924.** Newly revised medical-evangelism course (three months) began.
12. **February 27, 1925.** Dr. Fred E. Herzer, voted the first professor of hygiene.
13. **March 22, 1927.** Report to the Constituency: "During the past year the short course in medical missionary training has not been conducted." (Only three or four applicants for the program).

14. September 18, 1928. First research society in the CME initiated, the "Harveian Society."

15. March 20, 1930. Announcement: Beginning in the fall of 1930, the first students entering with 14 grades can complete their BS in Dietetics.

16. April 19, 1934. Board voted: Grant BS degrees to the first four dietetics students.

17. April 17, 1937. CME's first general accreditation (Northwestern Association of Secondary and Higher Schools), covering the Schools of Dietetics and of Nursing.

18. March 29, 1945. Announcement to Board: The Review and Herald Publishing Association gave $25,000 to fund research at Loma Linda. (Apparently, Loma Linda's first external funding for research.)

19. April 25, 1946. Board voted: To "look with favor" and "study" the establishment of a "School of Tropical Medicine" at Loma Linda.

20. January 1, 1947. CME employed Dr. Harold N. Mozar (under grant from Pacific Press) to work toward a School of Tropical and Preventive Medicine (STPM).

21. July 28–September 11, 1947: First course in "health evangelism and tropical hygiene," conducted at Loma Linda for mission appointees, Bible instructors, ministers, and other educators. This is first denominationally sponsored training of missionaries.

22. October 18, 1948. CME officially organized its STPM with Harold N. Mozar, as the director. STPM's first appropriation ($10,000) approved by the fall Council of the General Conference (October 26). Bruce Halstead employed as assistant director.

23. May 5, 1949. Board voted: Authorize STPM to employ Milton Murray as first public relations person in Seventh-day Adventist denomination (effective July 1).

24. June 9, 1950. Board voted: Approve $1,420 allowance to finance STPM's first summer course in tropical medicine in Mexico (July 30-September 6)

25. June 17, 1950. STPM received first grant from NIH, a co-operative project (research on poisonous fish) with Office of Naval Research.

26. July 24–August 4, 1950. Loma Linda hosted first "Institute of Scientific Studies for the Prevention of Alcoholism."

27. March 30, 1951. End of six-week course in parasitology and tropical hygiene for nurses. Offered by STPM and Christian Medical Council. (First course in the United States for nurses going to the tropics).

28. April 15, 1952. Board voted: To change name "School of Dietetics" to "School of Nutrition," with internship on Los Angeles campus designated as "Graduate School of Dietetics."

29. January 8, 1953: Board voted: Create "Council of Graduate Studies." Announcement: Graduate training available in nutrition and tropical medicine.

30. May 25, 1955. Board voted:
1. STPM become an integral part of CME
2. GC reinstate its annual appropriation ($30,000) to STPM

3. Health service (students and employees) to be utilized in teaching preventive medicine.

4. Mission appointees to receive instruction in hygiene. Training in tropical medicine for those going to tropical areas.

5. Discontinue fundraising in individual schools, centralizing it in University administration.

31. August 1956. CME Announcement: Research and assistance program for East Africa. 1. To strengthen program at Heri Hospital; 2. To encourage self-improvement in local Ha tribe.

32. November 1957. Announcement: Beginning of Adventist Health Studies. CME's researchers' three-year cancer study on California's 65,000 Adventists. Funded by NIH, led by Dr. Frank R. Lemon.

33. July 1958. Initiation of "student mission fellowships" in Mexico, Belize, Puerto Rico, and Monument Valley. Supervisors: Drs. Frank Lemon and John Peterson.

34. August 31, 1958. Bruce Halstead's resignation from STPM. (Set up his own research institute).

35. January 1960. Karl Fischer began construction of STPM Field Station at Heri Hospital. (Included school building, model village [student housing], and a duplex home for teachers.)

36. February 24, 1960. Western Association of Schools and Colleges (WASC) accredited CME.

37. December 15, 1960. Board voted: Rename STPM "division of public health and tropical medicine" (DPH&TM). Director, Harold Mozar.

38. March 1961. Announcement: Board approval for DPH&TM's MS degree in "health education," through Graduate School. (Beginning in September)

39. July 1, 1961. CME became Loma Linda University (LLU).

40. September 26, 1961. Board voted: Rename "School of Graduate Studies" as "The Graduate School."

41. February 15, 1962. Board authorization: Transfer School of Dietetics from Los Angeles to the Loma Linda campus. Rename "School of Dietetics" as "School of Nutrition and Dietetics" (April 26).

42. April 26, 1962. Board approval: First six candidates, MS degree in health education (Graduate School).

43. September 25, 26, 1962. Board decision to unite the medical school on one campus, at Loma Linda.

44. December 1962. LLU certified 11 African Adventist workers (from eight different tribes) as health education assistants after one academic year of practical training at Heri Hospital.

45. January 29, 1963. Board approved: Graduate curricula for health education and nutrition. Tropical public health curriculum referred for further study.

46. October 11, 1963. Announcement: "Executive physicals" at Loma Linda (Frank Lemon and Richard Walden). Predecessor of the Center for Health Promotion.

47. December 20, 1963. Completion of STPM's "research and assistance program." South Africa Division of Seventh-day Adventist took over public health training at Heri Hospital (continued affiliation with Loma Linda).

48. May 26, 1964. Board voted: Establishment of "division of nutrition and public health." To replace three entities: "School of Nutrition and Dietetics," "division of public health and tropical medicine," and the "department of preventive medicine and public health of the School of Medicine." To develop into a "School of Nutrition and Public Health."

49. August 25, 1964. Board voted: Implementation of new "division of nutrition and public health," (September 1, 1964), Mervyn G. Hardinge, director. Recognized as first step to LLU's "School of Public Health"

50. January 26, 1965. Board voted: "division of nutrition and public health" to be designated "division of public health (DPH)."

51. October 29–November 7, 1965. First Adventist live-in lifestyle program at Fontainbleau State Park, Louisiana, Jay L. Neil, director. P. William Dysinger (acting director, DPH), LLU's representative.

52. September 27, 1966. Board voted: Merger between "School of Nutrition and Dietetics" and "School of Public Health," effective after provisional SPH accreditation. A section of dietetics to be organized within SPH "department of nutrition."

53. February 8, 1967. Board voted: 1. DPH to become "School of Public Health" (SPH); Mervyn G. Hardinge, dean. 2. To combine "School of Nutrition and Dietetics" with the new SPH as its "department of nutrition and dietetics." 3. Hardinge also chair, "department of preventive medicine and public health" in School of Medicine.

54. June 23, 1967. Executive Board of the American Public Health Association granted full accreditation to LLU School of Public Health. The sixth professional school at Loma Linda and 15th SPH in the United States. Instruction began on July 1. LLU SPH voted in as 16th full member of the Association of Schools of Public Health (October).

55. December 19, 1967. Board voted: Authorization of eight separate departments in the SPH (effective July 1, 1968).

56. January 22, 1969. Razing of STPM building, originally "South Hall Laboratory." SPH offices and classrooms move to former Loma Linda Sanitarium (Nichol Hall). South Laboratory built (1919) for medical school lab space, then clinical lab and outpatient dispensary (1925). Home of STPM (since 1948) and SPH (since 1964).

57. September 14, 1970. SPH renamed "School of Health," emphasizing lifestyle programs of School.

58. September 1972. Beginning of new doctor of health science program, to train doctors in evaluation and promotion of health. (First graduates, May 1974.)

59. January 11, 1973. Announcement: LLU first to make physical fitness testing available to all its students

60. **June 27, 1973.** Board voted: Discontinuation of department of preventive medicine in School of Medicine.
61. **September 1973.** First SPH off-campus degree program teaching in Alberta, Canada (two courses offered).
62. **August 15, 1974.** Announcement by P. William Dysinger: Contract signed between LLU SPH and USAID (Department of State) to provide maternal and child health assistance to Tanzanian government. First such agreement negotiated by LLU or Adventist Church. Richard Hart, field director, for first two of seven-year program.
63. **January 30, 1975.** Organizational meeting of Students for International Medical Service (SIMS). "Mission" later substituted for "Medical."
64. **October 28, 1977.** Re-accreditation of SPH (maximum possible five years). LLU SPH recognized as the only church-oriented school of public health in the nation. Accrediting body commended SPH on commitment to its goals.
65. **March 20, 1980.** Announcement: SPH is offering MSPH degree program in international health to 150 students in the Inter-American Division of Seventh-day Adventist. Four sites: Haiti, Mexico/Costa Rica, Columbia/Puerto Rico, and Trinidad/Jamaica. Three languages: French, Spanish, and English.
66. **June 12, 1980.** Report on DHSc degree program (first graduates, 1974). Today, 80 percent of the 80 graduates have served in health science teaching, lifestyle related research, health promotion or health counseling. Fourteen of 80 posted overseas (13 in church mission programs). Thirty-seven of 66 in United States are employed by the Seventh-day Adventist Church.
67. **June 15, 1980.** First DrPH degree awarded to Terrell W. Zollinger (research in cancer epidemiology). Employed at Indiana University.
68. **April 9, 1981.** Kathleen K. Zolber, head, nutritional services, LLUMC and chair of dietetics, School of Allied Health Professions, was voted president-elect of American Dietetic Association (assumed presidency September 1982).
69. **May 16, 1983.** Board voted: Center for Health Promotion to be joint program between School of Public Health and School of Medicine.
70. **January 13, 1986.** Reorganization of School of Public Health. No more departments, only "programs" with individual program directors.
71. **July 1, 1986.** Department of preventive medicine re-established in School of Medicine by Board authorization: chair, Richard H. Hart.
72. **January 13, 1987.** Board voted: Consolidation of La Sierra and Loma Linda campuses in Loma Linda University. Then, Board voted consolidation plan be postponed. (May 19)
73. **August 24, 1987.** Board voted: Rename "School of Health" as "School of Public Health."
74. **January 11, 1988.** Board voted: 1. To unify current programs at La Sierra and Loma Linda (in marathon 11-hour session). 2. To postpone decision of structure of LLU (June 22, 1989). 3. To restructure LLU as single university, with dual organizational structure (August 28, 1989).

75. **December 20, 1988.** Announcement: SPH departments restored and departmental chairs named.

76. **March 22, 1989.** Announcement: LLU on two-year probation by WASC. Letter from the Council on Education for Public Health declared SPH interim report unacceptable (October). Another report required, May 1990.

77. **February 13, 1990.** Board voted: 1. Separation of Loma Linda and Riverside campuses (all previous actions rescinded). 2. Restructure the SPH under department of preventive medicine in School of Medicine (SM). (Public assumed Board had closed SPH.)

78. **April 2, 1990.** Board voted: 1. Restructure of SPH within SM (separate-School status to continue to 12/31/91). 2. Transfer administrative personnel, departments, programs from SPH to SM (May 19). 3. Merger announced as being complete (October 10).

79. **May 16, 1991.** Board voted: SPH to return to status of "a regular school within the University;" Richard Hart, dean. 2. DHSc degree reorganized as DrPH degree (in preventive care). 3. Previous public health programs in SM restored to SPH (December 12), program directors once again department chairs.

80. **March 1, 1992.** Announcement: WASC reaffirmed LLU's accreditation.

81. **May 19, 1992.** Board voted: Reaffirmation of support of SPH, including $500,000 to build up departments of environmental health and health administration.

82. **May 26, 1993.** WHO designated SPH a "Collaborating Center in Primary Health Care and Public Health Education."

83. **October 26, 1993.** CEPH awarded full accreditation to SPH (through December 1996).

84. **April 4, 1994.** Announcement: Ownership of medical facility at Norton AFB transferred to LLU. A large expansion of University's SAC program.

85. **February 4, 2001.** University Board voted: Richard H. Hart as first chancellor of LLU (inauguration October 24). Patricia Johnston appointed dean, SPH (July 18).

86. **August 31, 2003.** Ceremony at University of East Africa, Baraton, recognized 60 MPH graduates from 27 different African countries.

87. **April 30, 2004.** Grand opening of the geographic information systems laboratory, in the Del E. Webb Memorial Library. The LLU SPH, only school in the world to offer a BS in health geographics and maintain a geographic information systems laboratory.

88. **May 21, 2004.** Board voted: James L. Kyle II, dean, SPH, effective July 1, 2004.

Appendix III

Visions of the Future

This review of the exciting, inspiring history of public health at Loma Linda over the past 100 years has prompted me to look ahead. My dreams of the future of public health/preventive medicine at Loma Linda University are personal. Still, I hope that they will stimulate the interest of those who will deal with unfinished business in LLU's future.

1. I Dream of a Renewal of "Medical Evangelism" Training.

Loma Linda University owes an enormous debt of gratitude to its founding body, the Seventh-day Adventist Church. This organization has financially supplemented almost all public health endeavors at Loma Linda, both past and present. Indeed, the SPH could not exist without such support. Current faculty and students seriously owe it to themselves to study and fulfill CME/LLU's original mission.

That mission was to train people who would have the scientific expertise and ability to share the "good news" of both the gospel and abundant health to the world. In 1906, the College served two categories of people—medical evangelists and nurses. Ellen White wrote: "Thousands are to be qualified with all the ability of physicians to labor, not as physicians, but as medical missionary evangelists."[1]

Subsequently, many attempts were made to fulfill this mandate. By 1926, however, after strong efforts, the president admitted failure: "I regret to report that during the present school year no classes are being conducted for the special class of students whom we have called medical evangelistic or medical missionary students .... It appears there is so little demand for medical training outside of that furnished in the regular medical course, the nurses training course, and the dietitian training course, that it is impractical to arrange for such special courses at present."[2]

Sadly, CME never resumed this goal as formal course work.

In 1968, LLU School of Public Health undertook a new effort to train health evangelists in a program called "church health education." A special MSPH was prepared to train "ministers, church workers, and missionaries who anticipate a health emphasis in their activities."[3] New approaches to cities, public evangelism, and other such efforts were incorporated. A joint degree program with the Theological

Seminary at Andrews University enabled many, primarily ministers, to go through this training.

This second large effort to fulfill the original mandate failed. Andrews cancelled its participation (1980), and after 1985 interest at Loma Linda waned. Lack of activity doomed the idea to oblivion.

As early as 1938, Dr. Percy T. Magan, then CME president, pleaded for the life of the dream: "Now will you go back with me to the days when Ellen G. White walked this hill and remember her statement that we should train a few doctors and a large number of others with the qualifications of physicians, but without the legal qualifications. You know how in an early day here we tried very, very hard to get together classes to train them in medical ministry or medical evangelism .... We were unable to stem the tide that drove against us. We dropped the effort."

Magan concluded with this challenge:

"My dear friends, we are firmly of the opinion that every good word that God has ever spoken concerning this place will be fulfilled before the end. It looks to us as if a plan may be worked out ... whereby men going into the ministry may have some training in this place in a conjoint course which will unite medical ministry with the work of preaching the gospel. This is one thing which must be done before the end."[4]

This plan has never been implemented. My dream is that Magan's prophecy may yet be fulfilled in the public health program at Loma Linda.

2. I Dream of Using the Team Approach to Solving Health Problems.

I am convinced that team-work is the most powerful approach to public health work. All public health disciplines must be integrated in order to meet all of the important health needs of communities. Unfortunately, we find few good examples of public health disciplines working together, at Loma Linda or in any other place that I know of.

An early effort to combine the expertise of all faculty and students in the School of Public Health focused on a single problem: the treatment and prevention of coronary atherosclerosis. The outcome should have been a "conditioning center" or live-in lifestyle change center in a pleasant, resort type environment. A massive effort in both basic and applied research could have involved all of the Schools in the University. Heart disease as the number one cause of death in the United States and many other countries as well, deserved such an effort.[5]

This plan ran aground in 1966. I dream of another such effort being put forth.

Another opportunity for a team approach lies in the assessment and relief of major health problems among groups of people (ethnic populations, church congregations, and other well-defined communities, worldwide). Ideally, the study population would be located in Southern California with easy access for faculty and students from Loma Linda. Any such team-approach would begin with a detailed health needs assessment. It would be followed by setting goals and objectives, enumerating the resources needed, planning, and then implementing both basic research and action programs. Securing early community involvement would, of course, be crucial. Training local workers, supervision, and continuous evaluation would be an on-going part of the program.

Another approach for team effort would be the challenge of specific disease problems. For instance, an HIV/AIDS program could easily engage all the faculty and students. So, we examine AIDS. How do we define, control, prevent, or treat this plague to humanity? How it is spread and controlled in various cultures? Other than AIDS, there are many other diseases from which to choose—malaria, diabetes mellitus, hypertension, anxiety/depression, obesity, and other common serious degenerative diseases.

So I dream of what could be accomplished if all the resources of the School of Public Health were focused on solving one problem or working with the needs of one group of people. The results of such a serious effort could be breathtaking. The entire public health world would pay attention. Besides, imagine how such an exercise could truly unite faculty and students.

3. I Dream that Every Alumnus Will be a Teacher.

To teach others is the best way to learn. A basic fact of education, in fact. Almost every course taught in the SPH could deliberately prepare a student for this function. He/she would follow a simple outline and share knowledge at a layman's level. Groups sponsored by a local church, a civic group, an adult education organization, or a local community college—all could benefit.

The LLU SPH could provide a certificate of attendance. Alumni could be authorized to teach specific courses, following the guidelines set out by the distance learning office. In fact, any student who successfully completes a graduate course could be certified as a teacher of that subject to a lay audience.

The program could be a very satisfying outlet for many alumni, providing them with a supplementary income. At the same time, SPH would receive evaluation feedback on how well the teaching went. The costs of such a program could be covered by a fee charged by LLU for providing the certificate to those who satisfactorily complete the lay course.

I strongly believe that every graduate from the School of Public Health at Loma Linda should recognize him/herself as a teacher of others. In this way, LLU could enormously extend its outreach.

I dream that just such an opportunity might happen.

4. I Dream of International Public Health Coordination.

LLU and/or the Seventh-day Adventist Church now has public health training programs at the bachelor's degree or graduate level in Kenya, Mexico, Argentina, Chile, Peru,

Russia, the Philippines, and other places. The potential for new programs in Africa, India, and elsewhere indicates continuing and escalating interest in this kind of education.

Therefore, I foresee the urgent necessity of maintaining standardization and quality control for all Adventist public health training. At present, unity is maintained by the fact that most teachers have trained at Loma Linda, but this will undoubtedly change. Increasingly lectures and courses can become available on the Internet or on DVD's. This measure would improve the standard of public health education where few faculty are available to cover the many public health disciplines.

Included in this dream is a consortium of all Adventist institutions teaching public health. Several considerations emerge.

1. The General Conference or other respected co-ordination agency would supervise the consortium. (Prejudice of some against Loma Linda would preclude LLU dictating all programs and policies.)
2. Participating institutions would regularly share experiences and outlines by means of an e-mail network.
3. Teachers of the various public health disciplines would come together for annual workshops. Here they would learn from one another, finding ways to improve their didactic teaching and their practical fieldwork.
4. A three- or four-year rotation schedule might serve teachers of all public health disciplines—health education, health administration, nutrition, environmental health, tropical public health, lifestyle medicine, epidemiology/biostatistics, or other subject areas.
5. Place of meetings should rotate through a carefully planned schedule. Ideally, each school teaching public health would occasionally host the consortium in their own home institution.

Truly, unity and co-ordination is a rich dream!

5. I Dream of a Primary Health Care and Lifestyle Medicine Emphasis.

I envision the SPH helping people not only to recognize the importance of their own symptoms, but also to take responsibility for their individual and family health—physical, mental, and spiritual. I hope for a paradigm shift by physicians' emphasizing diagnosis, treatment of individual signs, symptoms, or diseases. Rather, they would help people improve their lifestyle, wisely choosing ways to increase their immunity and improve health and happiness.

Such an educational approach includes emphasizing integrated community development. Local communities could organize themselves to care for the majority of their primary health care. Obviously, a good referral system and training to recognize serious signs would have to be in place. Also, a well-developed and organized home health care and support system is required.

Philosophically, this approach applies everywhere, both in the United States and in poorer countries. Such an organization could do much to replace the Adventist hospital-based medical care system. Since hospitals increasingly find themselves in difficult financial and management situations, I believe this to be a very good proposition. Such a program holds promise of significantly lowering the high costs of health care. The dream of better living and higher levels of health is a large one.

6. I Dream of a Center for Tropical Medicine and Foreign Service Training.

The direct predecessor to the LLU's School of Public Health was the CME School of Tropical and Preventive Medicine (1947). It stood as only the second tropical medicine school in the United States. LLU now works directly with more foreign students and has affiliations (through the Adventist Church) in more foreign countries than any other SPH. Ironically, it does not have any center in which one can obtain basic information on diseases occurring in the poorest countries of the world. No single department or school within the University exists where tropical medicine and or tropical public health information is easily available.

I dream that LLU should support a specialist in tropical medicine or tropical public health in the School of Public Health. That person would have at least three tasks:

1. To coordinate and help supervise all efforts to prepare health professionals to work in the poor areas of the world.
2. To oversee the examination services for persons preparing for foreign service or returning from the developing world.
3. To otherwise assist all LLU schools and programs preparing persons for mission service in Africa, Asia, Latin America, or other lesser developed countries.

My dream also includes a material component. A facility would be built to include an office, special laboratory, and examination rooms. The library would contain the principal tropical medicine monographs and journals. Also demonstration slides of human parasites and vector borne disease organisms, along with area information, teaching videos, or other training materials. All kinds of appropriate resource material could be brought together in one place, together with suggestions for self study. What a boon for health workers doing research or for those seeking answers to specific questions relating to tropical disease and cross-cultural medicine.

With malaria and other so-called tropical diseases increasing, and the dangers of new and emerging exotic diseases such as SARS and avian influenza threatening the world, Loma Linda needs to become a place for advice, consultation, prevention, treatment, and training. LLU ought to be able to deal with all of these health problems. I dream of Loma Linda University being recognized as pre-eminent in this area of expertise.

7. I Dream of a Health Museum Connected with the Center for Health Promotion.

One of the original objectives of the founding dean of the SPH at Loma Linda was for an interactive health museum. He imagined a place where the basic health sciences and recommended lifestyle practices would be displayed—and displayed in such a manner as to make learning attractive to the public.

Such a museum would serve several purposes:

1. A significant display of the Creation model for human life and development, along with such distinctive beliefs as the Sabbath, and more.
2. A presentation of the historical background of developments at Loma Linda.
3. An exhibit showing the cultural differences that affect health in many different people-groups around the world.[6]
4. An environment conducive to learning new health philosophy and practices—classrooms, seminar rooms, and multi-media rooms.

Such a facility might be directly associated with a new Center for Health Promotion where state of the art health assessments and risk reduction programs could be on-going.

Inevitably, the health museum would be an attraction for the entire Southern California region and be a place of learning for scheduled elementary and high school classes and other groups as well as a teaching laboratory for students in the School of Public Health.

A very pleasant location to be considered for the building would be the site of the original hotel-sanitarium. Included would be the space over the area where the original stairs came up the hill from the railway station. A parking garage and access for the public could be at the bottom of the hill. The staff and student entrance could be at the top of the hill, into the top floor of the multi-story edifice built over the hillside.

Would not this dream make the Hill Beautiful once more?

I have shared these my dreams in order to stimulate readers to dream their own dreams. Others may have better dreams than mine. Maybe mine even seem impractical to some. Nonetheless, all who have connections with Loma Linda's School of Public Health should brainstorm creative ideas. Alumni, faculty, and students are all in this together.

Then, to be sure, God will lead into new methods that can bless mankind and foster His kingdom of love and peace on earth.

[1] E. G. White: *Loma Linda Messages*, p. 15.

[2] "CME Annual Report of the President," *The Medical Evangelist*, April 7, 1938, p. 2.

[3] *University Scope*, September 11, 1968.

[4] "Report of CME President Magan to the Constituency", *The Medical Evangelist*, April 7, 1938, p. 2.

[5] "Health Sciences Advancement Award Proposal," prepared in 1966 by P. W. Dysinger and the faculty of the DPH of LLU.

[6] Ideas for such an interactive museum were included in a doctoral thesis by early HLED professor Harold Shull. His research included visits to many such museums in the United States and a WHO sponsored travel fellowship to study such museums in Europe.

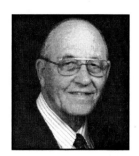

About the Author

Paul William Dysinger (CME '55) MD, MPH

P. William (Bill) Dysinger grew up in his home state of Tennessee with his eyes fixed on doing medical missionary work in Peru. To this end, he studied Spanish in high school at Madison, Tennessee and again during his pre-medical study at Southern Missionary College. He graduated in the first accredited senior college class at SMC in 1951. He began medical studies at Loma Linda that same year and while still in medical school, he helped stimulate the last STPM tropical medicine field trip to Mexico. Useful preparation for life and work in Peru, as he saw it. Then, his career took some other turns.

After a general internship at Washington Adventist Hospital in Maryland, Dysinger fulfilled his military obligation with two years of service with the United States Public Health Service working for Native Americans in Montana and Arizona—the Blackfeet and Navajo/Hopis.

Afterward, he transferred to the U.S. State Department for training in the Foreign Service Institute. In September 1958, he and his bride of four months, Yvonne Minchin, flew to Phnom Penh, Cambodia, where they served two years with the American Embassy. During this time in diplomatic service, they visited mission hospitals and stations in more than 60 countries around the world.

The Dysingers brought this experience and their enthusiasm to the founding of the international health program at Loma Linda. Peru as a destination receded into the distance. As he spent most of his fifty years of international health service in Africa and Asia, his knowledge of Spanish slipped away.

Dr. Dysinger's formal connection with Loma Linda began in 1961 when he worked with Frank Lemon in the first Adventist mortality study. (His personal research lay in the epidemiologic analysis of emphysema and auto accident fatalities among Adventists.) Later in that same year, he entered Harvard School of Public Health where he completed an interdepartmental MPH, with emphasis on health administration and the teaching of preventive medicine.

In the summer of 1962, he and his family traveled to Tanganyika (now Tanzania). They spent the next two years directing the new community health-worker training at Heri Hospital in the highlands above Kigoma and Ujiji. He returned to Loma Linda in 1964 in time to help Dr. Mervyn G. Hardinge in the initial planning for the School of Public Health. During Hardinge's sabbatical in 1965–66, Dysinger served as acting director of the division of public health, and working with Elder Jay Lee Neil, he helped launch Adventist lifestyle change programs.

Dysinger served as the associate dean of the School of Public Health for academic affairs and international health during its first fourteen years (including its first three accreditation cycles). At Loma Linda he held several positions: In the dean's office and as chair of four different departments (health science in the School of Allied Health Professions, and tropical health, health administration, and international health in the School of Public Health). He also assisted the beginnings of the preventive medicine residency in the School of Medicine and helped to initiate preventive medicine in the Veterans Administration hospital system.

While headquartered at Loma Linda for 28 years, Dysinger kept his hands active in international health projects in Tanzania, New Guinea, Pakistan, Singapore, Honduras, the Philippines, Lebanon, Norway, and elsewhere. From Loma Linda, he transferred to the General Conference of Seventh-day Adventists headquarters in 1988 where he served five years as the first physician senior health advisor for ADRA International. He concentrated on projects in more than 40 countries, with special emphasis on child survival projects.

Since retirement in 1992, the Dysingers have maintained relations with Loma Linda University, where he is listed as associate dean emeritus of the School of Public Health. He has also served long-term on the Boards of Adventist Frontier Missions, Adventist Southeast Asia Projects, and other community and humanitarian organizations. He has otherwise kept busy authoring books and articles, consulting overseas, and working on their 180 acre farm located in middle Tennessee (near where he was born). He and Yvonne keep active in local church and community programs. In 1998–99, they worked with ADRA in Yemen, where he was volunteer country director.

Increasingly the Dysingers are involved with their four children—Edwin, Wayne, John, and Janelle, their spouses, and fourteen grandchildren and one great-grandson. Their son Wayne is now back in Loma Linda where he serves as chair of the LLU department of preventive medicine in the School of Medicine and works closely with the LLU School of Public Health. The other Dysinger children live near Bill and Yvonne, and they are involved with their parents in many projects and programs to serve needy people both locally and abroad.

During the years 2002–2006, Bill and Yvonne spent much time at Loma Linda doing the research necessary to complete this first history of public health, medical evangelism, and community outreach during the first 100 years of the College of Medical Evangelists and Loma Linda University. They found God's providential leading in helping Loma Linda to take "health to the public" a fascinating and rewarding investigation.

Their research leads to the prayer that the vision to make and keep man whole will remain strong in the hearts and minds of both staff and students at Loma Linda as long as time shall last.